ECG Diagnosis Made Easy

ECG Diagnosis Made Easy

Romeo Vecht FRCP, FACC, FESC

Consultant Cardiologist
The Wellington Hospital
London NW8 9LE
UK
Honorary Visiting Consultant
Royal Brompton Hospital
London SW3 6NP
UK

MARTIN DUNITZ

© 2001 Martin Dunitz Ltd, a member of the Taylor & Francis group

First published in the United Kingdom in 2001
by Martin Dunitz Ltd, The Livery House, 7–9 Pratt Street, London NW1 0AE

Tel.:   +44 (0)20 7482 2202
Fax.:   +44 (0)20 7267 0159
E-mail: info.dunitz@tandf.co.uk
Website: http://www.dunitz.co.uk

Although every effort has been made to ensure that drug doses and other
information are presented accurately in this publication, the ultimate respon-
sibility rests with the prescribing physician. Neither the publishers nor the
authors can be held responsible for errors or for any consequences arising
from the use of information contained herein. For detailed prescribing information or instructions on the use of any product or procedure discussed
herein, please consult the prescribing information or instructional material
issued by the manufacturer.

A CIP record for this book is available from the British Library.

ISBN 1-85317-721-0

Distributed in the United States by:
Blackwell Science Inc.
Commerce Place, 350 Main Street
Malden MA 02148
Tel.: +1-800-215-100

Distributed in Canada by:
Login Brothers Book Company
324 Salteaux Crescent
Winnipeg, Manitoba R3J 3T2
Tel.: +1-204-224-4068

Distributed in Brazil by:
Ernesto Reichmann Distribuidora de Livros, Ltda
Rua Coronel Marques 335
Tatuape 03440-000, Sao Paulo

Composition by Scribe Design, Gillingham, Kent, UK
Printed and bound in Italy by Printer Trento S.r.l.

Contents

	Introduction	*ix*
1	*Basic principles*	*1*
2	*Ischaemic (coronary) heart disease*	*9*
3	*Conduction impairment*	*63*
4	*Rhythm disturbances*	*105*
5	*Hypertrophy*	*161*
6	*Cardiomyopathies and autoimmune disorders*	*169*
7	*Pericarditis, myocarditis and metabolic disorders*	*179*
8	*Pacemakers, ICDs (implantable cardiac defibrillators) and cardioversion*	*187*
9	*Mixed ECG quizzes*	*205*
	Further reading	*225*
	Drug regimen tables	*227*
	Index	*231*

This book is dedicated to my teachers who
have stimulated me to understand

Borné dans sa nature, infini dans ses voeux
L'homme est un Dieu tombé, qui se souvient des cieux

Lamartine, 19th Century

Introduction

This book is intended primarily for those who want to acquire an understanding of electrocardiography. Therefore I have attempted to keep it simple, so as to explain the basic concept of the electrocardiogram; only a few references have been included to tempt further reading.

The illustrations were chosen to cover a wide spectrum of ECG pathologies with an emphasis on changes observed in real tracings. I have added short historical notes when appropriate and a therapeutic appendage for rapid reference.

Electrocardiography is the ability to recognise electric patterns based on sound scientific principles. It has vast applications in the fields of cardiology, cardiac surgery and general medicine. The electrocardiogram must be seen as a support to clinical diagnostic skill and not as a primary decision making instrument.

I have enjoyed producing this book, based on the belief that the art of teaching should be as pleasurable as the practice of medicine. I hope that my efforts will prove beneficial, stimulating and as enjoyable to read as they were to compile.

R Vecht
London

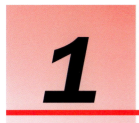

Basic principles

Electrical impulses in the heart

Electrical impulses are required to synchronise the four pumping chambers. The atria are electrically isolated from the ventricles by a fibrous atrioventricular separation. The impulse originates in the sino-atrial (SA) node, travels across the atrial musculature towards the atrioventricular (AV) node, thence down through the bundle of His to the ventricles via the right and left bundles and into the Purkinje system (Figure 1). The SA node has an inherent rate of approximately 70 beats per minute and is under autonomic and chemical hormonal influence. The inherent rate of the AV node is lower, at 60 beats per minute, and the ventricles will beat in isolation at approximately 40 or less beats per minute. The electrical impulse, having reached the ventricular musculature, then travels outwards from the endocardium to the epicardial surface. The electrical current is produced by a

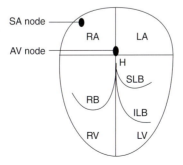

Figure 1: Electrical conduction through the heart. *From the sinoatrial node across the atrial musculature, the impulse reaches the atrioventricular node. It proceeds downwards through the bundle of His, then simultaneously to the right ventricle, through the right bundle and to the left ventricle through the two left bundles (termed anterior and posterior, or superior and inferior). Finally from endocardium to epicardium, the Purkinje system conducts the tail-end impulses. SA = sinoatrial node; AV = atrioventricular node; H = bundle of His; RV = right ventricle; LV = left ventricle; RB = right bundle; RA = right atrium; LA = left atrium; SLB = superior left bundle; ILB = inferior left bundle.*

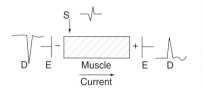

Figure 2: Muscle depolarisation. *When stimulated, the muscle develops a negative charge. An electrode facing the oncoming current will record an upright (positive) deflection. The current moving away inscribes a downward (negative) signal. Halfway between the two, the deflection is diphasic. D = deflection; E = electrode; – = negative; + = positive; S = stimulus.*

change of ionic forces from positive at rest to negative when activated (Figure 2).

Positioning electrodes for electrocardiography

The electrocardiogram consists of 12 electrodes placed around the heart. For mathematical purposes, the heart is at the centre of a triangle (Figure 3).

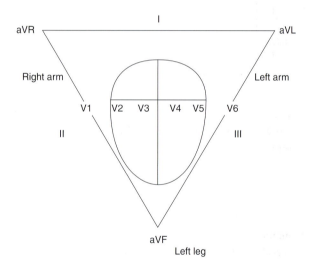

Figure 3: Position of electrodes around the heart. *Schematic representation of 12 leads (electrodes) placed around the heart.*

The electrode placements are designated as follows:

- **the three limb leads:** lead I joins the right and left arms, lead II connects the right arm and left leg and lead III joins the left arm and left leg.
- **the three augmented leads:** aVR is positioned facing the heart from the right arm, aVL from the left arm and aVF from the left foot. These electrodes are placed in a frontal plane.

- **the precordial leads (V1–V6):** these are placed on the front of the thorax and record horizontal impulses.

Topography of impulses

The conventional nomenclature is illustrated in Figure 4.

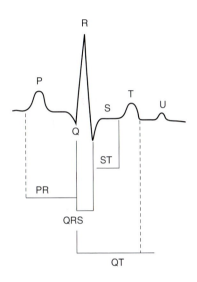

Figure 4: Normal ECG recording. *This denotation was introduced by Einthoven. The U wave is often not discernible. P = atrial depolarisation; QRS = ventricular depolarisation; T = ventricular repolarisation; U = either represents after-potentials of the ventricular myocardium or repolarisation of the Purkinje fibers. The PR interval represents the time taken from atrial to ventricular depolarisation. The ST segment should be isoelectric. The QT interval is the time taken from ventricular depolarisation to repolarisation.*

P can be positive or negative, Q is always negative, R is always positive, S is always negative and T can be either. U wave is upright; when inverted indicates ischaemia.

Physiological measurements

- PR interval = 0.12–0.2 s (120–200 ms)
- QRS duration = 0.06–0.1 s (60–100 ms)
- QT interval = 0.30–0.46 s (300–460 ms)

for heart rates varying between 45 to 115 beats per minute. The QT interval lengthens with bradycardia and shortens with tachycardia.

The atria

The SA node discharges from right to left. This is recorded as the P wave, which represents atrial depolarisation leading to atrial contraction (Figure 5). The repolarisation of the atria is lost in the QRS complex. The P wave will be inscribed as positive in leads facing the incoming signal (aVF, III and V6) and as negative in leads from which the current is moving away (aVR and V1).

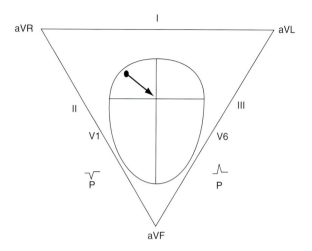

Figure 5: The P wave vector. *The P wave impulse travels from right to left. Leads facing the incoming signal (III, aVF and V6) will record a positive trace. Negative deflections appear in aVR and V1, the impulse being carried away from these sites.*

The ventricles

The QRS complex represents ventricular contraction, i.e. depolarisation. The complex consists of an **initial** septal activation followed by the major ventricular signal. Septal activation is from left to right, so that the leads facing the oncoming signal (II, aVF and V1) will record a positive trace R; lead V6 will record a negative trace Q (Figure 6).

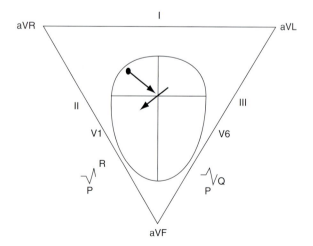

Figure 6: Septal activation. *The initial QRS activation results from the electrical impulse stimulating the interventricular septum through the bundle of His. The initial deflection will be positive in lead V1 and negative in lead V6.*

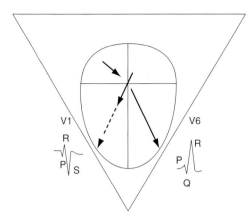

Figure 7: Ventricular activation. *The main vector (an electrical force that has both magnitude and direction) travels from right to left (RV currents are dwarfed by the thicker left ventricular musculature). Positive tracings are observed in leads III and V6 and a negative tracing is recorded from lead V1.*

The **main** ventricular activation affecting the left ventricle moves from right to left (Figure 7). This comprises all of the signals activating the left ventricle (the right ventricular currents are dwarfed by the left). Again, electrodes facing the oncoming current (e.g. leads III and V6) will record a positive wave, and those carrying the impulse away (e.g. V1) will record a negative wave.

Repolarisation of the ventricle gives rise to the T wave, which usually follows the QRS complex.

The electrical axis

Each ECG lead has a positive and a negative terminal. The three standard limb leads, I, II and III, are illustrated in Figure 8.

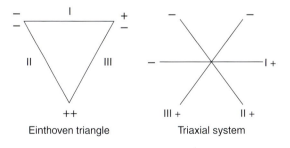

Einthoven triangle   Triaxial system

Figure 8: The three standard (limb) leads. *The Einthoven triangle translated into a triaxial system shows the positive and negative terminals of each lead.*

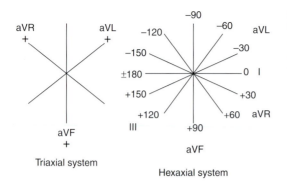

Figure 9: Standard and augmented leads. *Combination of all 12 leads showing polarity and degrees within a circle.*

The augmented leads are aVR, aVL and aVF. Here each limb lead has a positive terminal, the negative pole being connected to all three limb electrodes. The sum of the three limb leads equals zero potential, so the augmented leads have a positive terminal and a negative terminal at zero potential.

Using the hexaxial system (Figure 9), one is able to calculate the mean P, QRS or T wave axis.

The mean frontal QRS electrical axis is the one to concentrate on. The depolarisation of the ventricles (QRS) can be represented by a mean vector running from right to left. The maximum deflection in an ECG lead will represent a force running parallel to this lead. Thus considering an example in which lead II shows a maximum positive deflection, the axis will be +60° (Figure 10).

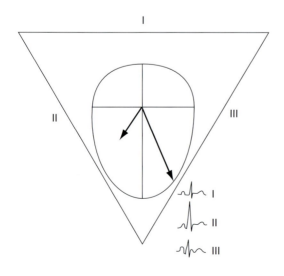

Figure 10: The mean vector of left ventricular depolarisation. *Lead II is the closest parallel to the mean vector of depolarisation. It shows the greatest deflection and an axis of +60°.*

a)   b)

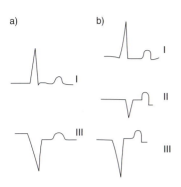

Figure 11: Left (superior) electrical axis deviation. A: *A left (superior) axis deviation is present when the main vectors in leads I and III move away from each other.* **B:** *When lead II is also negative (−30°), the trace is described as showing a 'pathological' left axis deviation and represents left ventricular problems.*

To keep things even simpler: if the vectors in leads I and III move away from one another, this represents left axis deviation (LAD). If, in addition, lead II is negative and the axis points to −30° or more, the trace is described as showing pathological left axis deviation. Left axis deviation indicates an abnormality of the left ventricle caused by numerous pathological entities.

If the vectors in leads I and III point towards one another this is known as right axis deviation (RAD) and denotes right-sided problems (Figure 12).

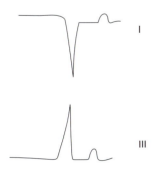

Figure 12: Right (inferior) electrical axis deviation. *The main deflections in leads I and III point towards one another. This indicates right-sided problems.*

LAD is present when the axis moves from 0 to −120° (i.e. it is superior) and RAD is present when the range is from +90 to +180 (i.e. it is inferior).

NB: LAD is also known as left anterior hemiblock, and RAD as left posterior hemiblock.

Historical notes

A Von Koellitzer (1817–1905) Swiss physiologist. First demonstrated muscular contraction associated with an electrical current.

AD Waller (1856–1922) Physiologist, St Mary's Hospital London, UK. Demonstrated electrical activity preceding cardiac contraction.

W Einthoven (1860–1927) Physiologist, Leiden, The Netherlands. Introduced PQRST nomenclature and string galvanometer.

W His (1863–1934) Professor of Medicine, Basel, Switzerland. Demonstrated the bundle named after him.

JE Purkinje (1787–1869) Professor of Physiology, Prague, Czechoslovakia. Discovered fibre formation beneath mucous membrane of the heart without recognising physiological significance.

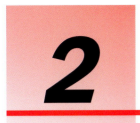

2 Ischaemic (coronary) heart disease

Atheromatous narrowing of the coronary arteries is a frequent pathological finding in the developed world. Stenosis and/or occlusion of a coronary artery leads to ischaemia and/or infarction of myocardial tissue with characteristic ECG changes.

Non Q wave infarction (subendocardial)

When the infarct spares some muscle, a non Q wave infarction results. Since blood flows from the epicardium to the endocardium, the latter is more vulnerable to ischaemia, being subjected to greater contractile forces. Ischaemic muscle produces a current of injury; healthy muscle has a positive charge which turns negative when stimulated. The baseline of the electrocardiogram thereby becomes depressed. During depolarisation, when the healthy muscle becomes negatively charged, no current flows. As the electrical signal returns to baseline this leads to elevation of the ST segment in electrodes facing the injured muscle. Thus a non Q wave infarct (also known as a subendocardial infarct), is characterised by ST elevation in the leads facing the damage. Conversely, ST depression is seen in leads facing the uninjured surface (Figure 13). Repolarisation is abnormal and gives rise to inverted T waves.

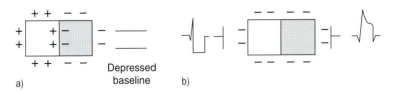

Figure 13: Current of injury. A: *The shaded area is ischaemic and becomes negatively charged. The ECG shows a depression of the baseline. **B:** During depolarisation the residual healthy muscle becomes negatively charged. No current flows. The baseline returns to normal and the ST segment appears elevated. The lead facing the injured muscle shows ST segment elevation. The lead facing the uninjured portion inscribes ST segment depression.*

Q Wave infarction (transmural, full thickness)

Q waves are seen when the entire wall of the ventricle is infarcted (a full thickness or transmural infarction). Three surfaces of the heart can be damaged separately: anterior, inferior (diaphragmatic) or true posterior (Figure 14). Infarcted tissue carries no electrical charge. The ECG electrode picks up electrical impulses travelling towards it through a 'dead window'.

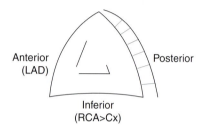

Figure 14: The three areas of myocardial infarction. *The anterior surface of the myocardium is supplied by the left anterior descending (LAD) artery. The inferior surface obtains its supply essentially from the right coronary artery (RCA) and occasionally from the circumflex (Cx) artery.*

Anterior myocardial infarction

Leads facing the infarct will record negative vectors (Q waves). As the main left ventricular vector that moves from right to left has been obliterated, negative vectors will be seen, inscribing Q waves on the ECG. These negative vectors result from 'unopposed' forces, that is septal and right ventricular depolarisation seen through the 'dead window' (Figure 15). Q waves are seen in leads I and aVL and V1–V6, depending on the extent of the damage. Q waves in leads V1–V3 indicate an anteroseptal infarct; in leads V3–V6 they indicate an anterolateral infarct, and in leads V1–V6 they signal extensive myocardial infarction (ECGs 1–30).

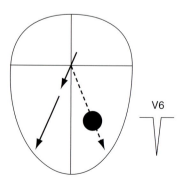

Figure 15: Anterior infarction. *Leads facing the infarcted territory pick up unopposed forces moving away through the non-conducting 'window', e.g. Q waves in V6.*

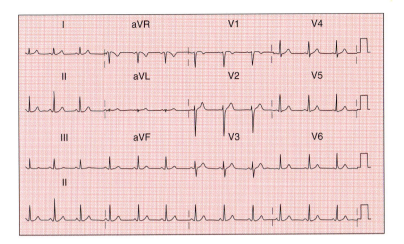

ECG 1: *Normal trace (LG; 24/4/98).*

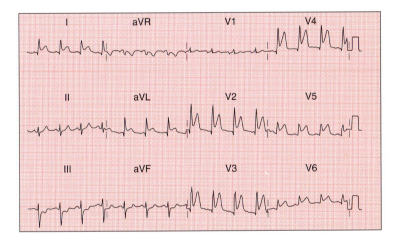

ECG 2: *Acute anterior infarction. ST elevation in leads I, aVL and V2–V6 (AN; 15/9/85).*

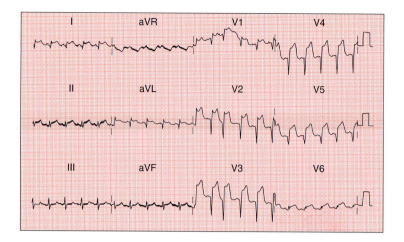

ECG 3: *The same patient 3 days later. Q waves are apparent in leads I, aVL and V1–V5. ST elevation is still present (AN; 18/9/85).*

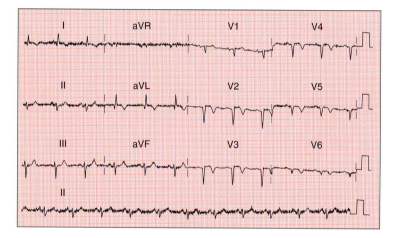

ECG 4: *Two years later the ST segments are back to baseline but Q waves are seen in leads I, aVL and V1–V6 with T wave inversions (AN; 6/2/87).*

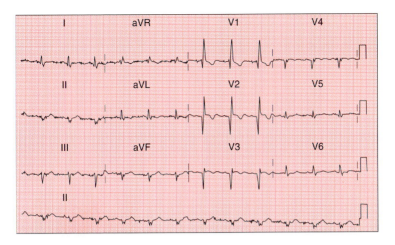

ECG 5: *Eleven years later the patient has developed right bundle branch block. The anteroseptal Q waves remain. Residual ST elevation in leads V2 and V3 are indicative of left ventricular aneurysm (AN; 25/11/98).*

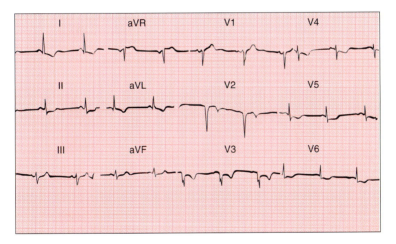

ECG 6: *Q wave anteroseptal infarct with widespread ST depression (MB; 3/10/79).*

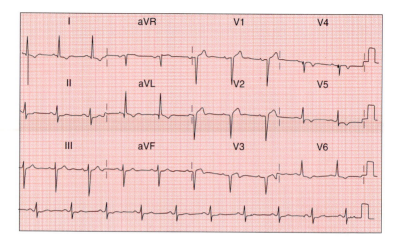

ECG 7: *The same patient 19 years later. The ECG has a very similar pattern, with fewer ST segment depressions. The patient was treated conservatively (NB; 29/6/98).*

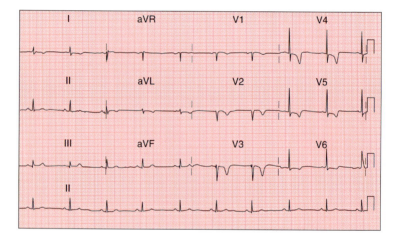

ECG 8: *Young male patient with acute anteroseptal infarction (CA; 4/6/98).*

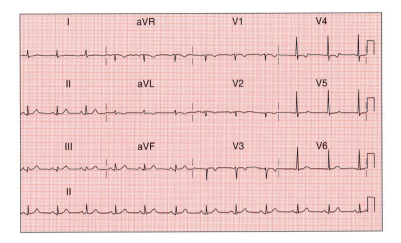

ECG 9: *This trace was recorded soon after successful angioplasty and stent insertion in LAD (CA; 19/6/98).*

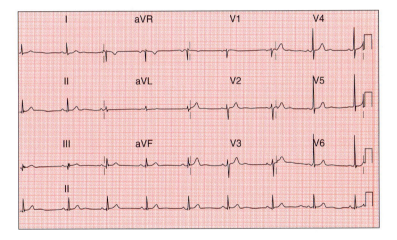

ECG 10: *After 3 months, the patient made a full recovery (CA; 28/9/98).*

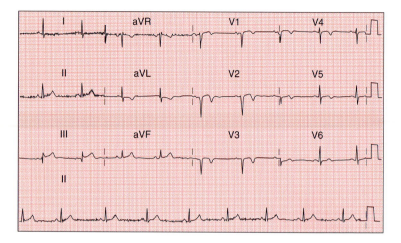

ECG 11: *Young male patient with anteroseptal Q wave infarction. He underwent a successful bypass operation (MG; 15/10/93).*

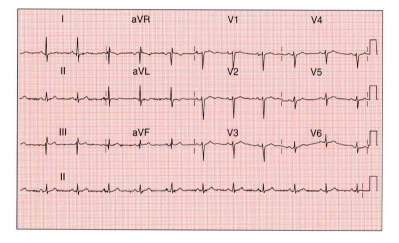

ECG 12: *After 6 years the only remaining abnormality is mild T wave inversion in lead aVL. R wave progression over the precordium has not fully recovered (MG; 22/9/99).*

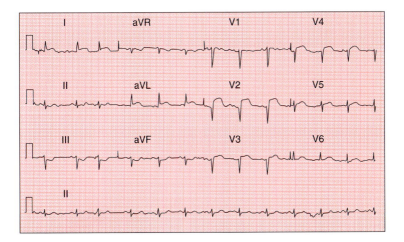

ECG 13: Widespread Q wave acute anterior infarction. ST segment elevation is present in leads I, aVL and V2–V5 with Q waves in lead V2 and reciprocal changes (ST segment depression) in leads III and aVF (TB; 30/7/99).

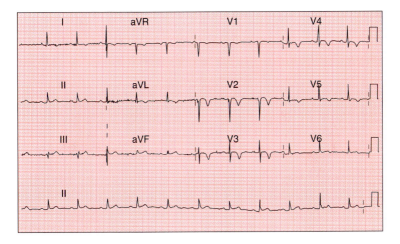

ECG 14: This 43-year-old male suffered severe chest pain after cycling. He had an anteroseptal infarct. The LAD artery was successfully ballooned and stented (AF; 12/4/99).

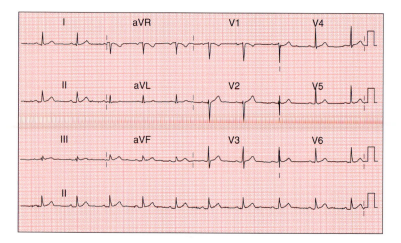

ECG 15: *The same patient was asymptomatic 5 months later. Minimal Q waves are visible in lead V2 only. The patient made a full recovery (AF; 21/9/99).*

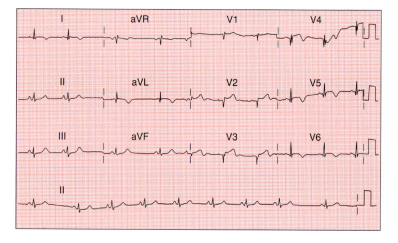

ECG 16: *Acute anteroseptal infarction (AR; 2/10/95).*

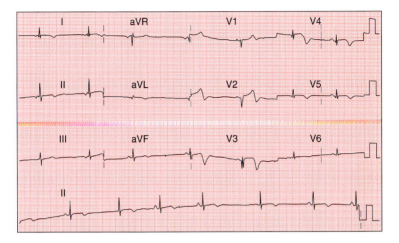

ECG 17: *More profound ischaemic changes are visible in leads V2 and V3, T wave inversions. These changes occurred 24 hours later, suggesting extension of the infarct (AR; 3/10/95).*

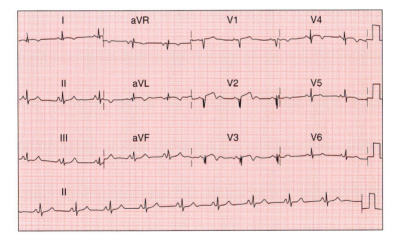

ECG 18: *There are fewer T wave inversions—a sign of recovery—2 days later (AR; 5/10/95).*

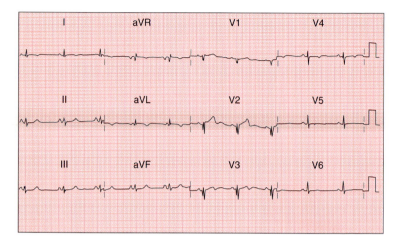

ECG 19: *Further improvement is evident 3 days after infarction (AR; 8/10/95).*

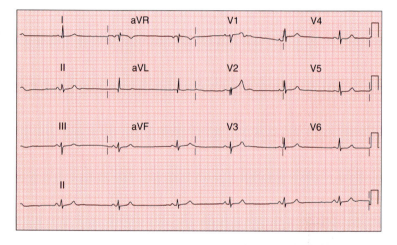

ECG 20: *Three years later, residual Q waves are visible in lead V2. ST segment elevation is present, possibly indicating a localised LV aneurysm. The patient underwent angioplasty to the left anterior descending artery soon after admission (AR; 7/10/98).*

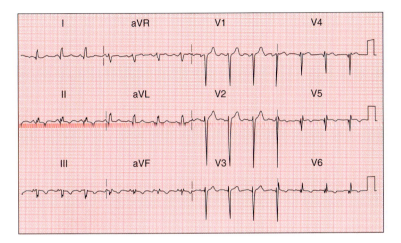

ECG 21: *Pre-intervention ECG. There is reduced R wave progression in leads V4–V5 (Mr P; 22/5/98).*

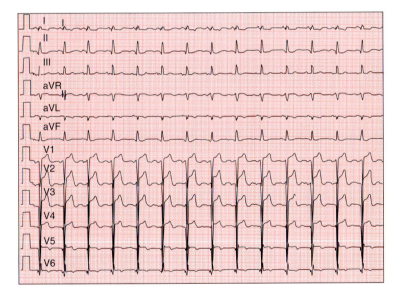

ECG 22: *During stent implantation. Marked ST segment elevation in leads V1–V5 during occlusion of the left anterior descending artery. The patient made a full recovery (Mr P; 22/5/98).*

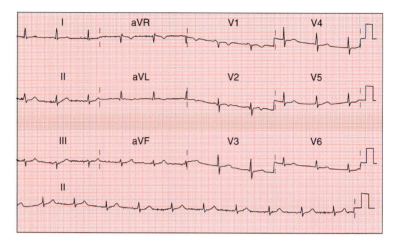

ECG 23: Patient with previous bypass surgery. Minor T wave changes are present in leads aVL and V2 (LG; 5/5/98).

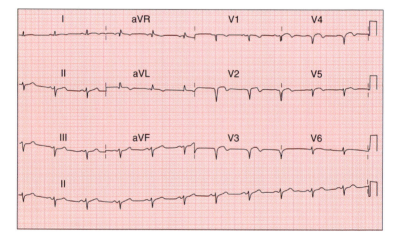

ECG 24: Acute anterior infarction caused by a blocked LAD vein graft was demonstrated at cardiac catheterisation 4 months later (LG; 22/9/98).

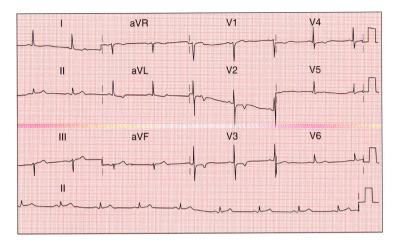

ECG 25: *This 57-year-old patient presented with unstable angina. Ischaemic changes (T wave inversions) are noted in the anteroseptal leads (I, aVL, V2, V3, V4) (SM; 13/3/93).*

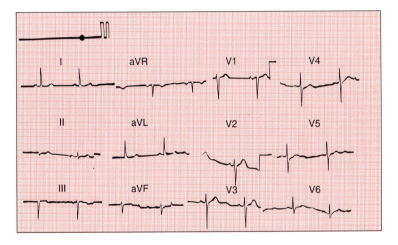

ECG 26: *After successful angioplasty, all changes returned to normal (SM; 24/13/93).*

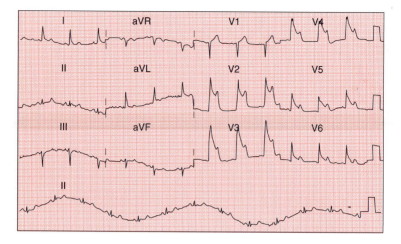

ECG 27: *The patient experienced further angina 3 months later. Angioplasty resulted in total occlusion of the left anterior descending artery, with marked ST segment elevations in leads V2–V6. Emergency bypass surgery was performed the same day (SM; 15/6/93).*

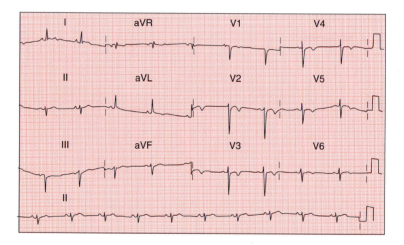

ECG 28: *Three days later, residual ischaemic changes are visible in leads V2–V5 (SM; 18/6/93).*

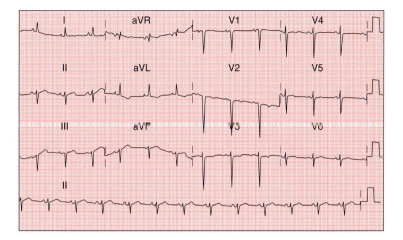

ECG 29: *Further improvement, but Q waves are visible in leads V1 and V2 (SM; 22/6/93).*

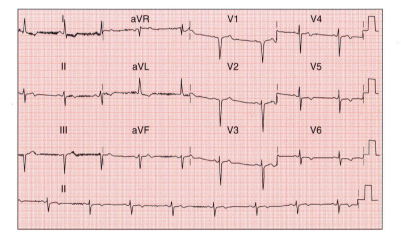

ECG 30: *After 5 years, the patient is well, but permanent 'ischaemic' changes are visible anterolaterally. Q waves are visible only in lead V1, indicating regenerating healthy muscle (SM; 18/5/98).*

Inferior myocardial infarction

The unopposed right-sided vectors (inferior window) show up as Q waves in the inferior leads—that is leads II, III and aVF (Figure 16 and ECGs 31-39).

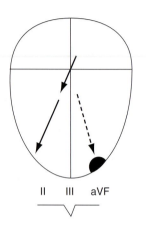

Figure 16: Inferior infarction. *Here the Q waves are seen in the inferior leads (II, III, aVF).*

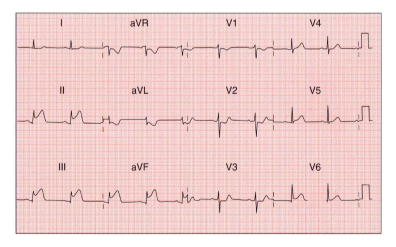

ECG 31: *Acute inferior infarction. ST segment elevations are present in leads II, III and aVF. Reciprocal changes are present in leads aVR, aVL, V1 and V2 (JB; 12/10/98).*

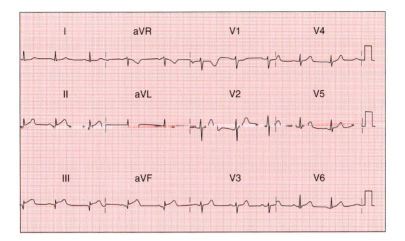

ECG 32: *There is rapid resolution after administration of intravenous thrombolysin (JB; 12/10/98).*

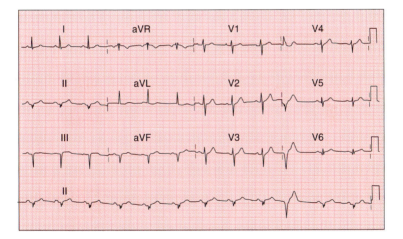

ECG 33: *Several hours later, Q waves are seen in leads II, III and aVF (JB; 12/10/98).*

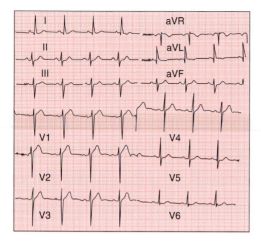

ECG 34: *Normal trace (AL; 14/9/70).*

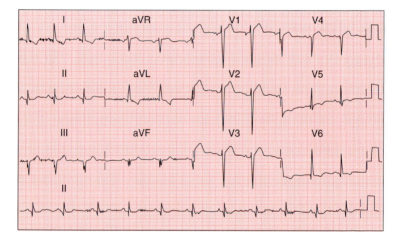

ECG 35: *The same patient suffered inferior infarction 16 years later. There are Q waves in leads II, III and aVF, and T inversions in the anterior lateral leads. The patient underwent bypass surgery (AL; 3/12/86).*

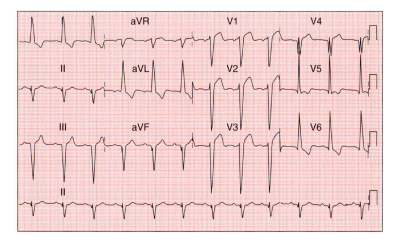

ECG 36: *After another 12 years, the patient has a left bundle branch block. Q waves are still visible in leads II, III and aVF (AL; 2/2/98).*

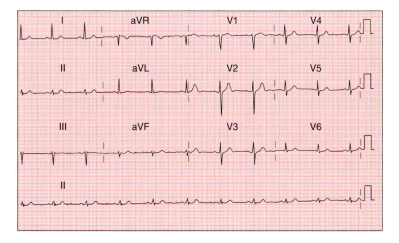

ECG 37: *Normal trace (ED; 28/1/98).*

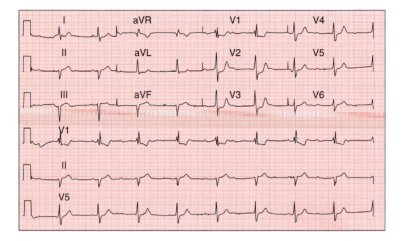

ECG 38: *Seven months later, the ECG indicates recent inferior infarction. There are Q waves in leads II, III and aVF. Reciprocal changes (ST segment depressions) are visible in leads V2 and V3. Lead V1 shows AV dissociation, suggesting complete heart block. P waves and QRS complexes are not connected, indicating conduction defects commonly seen with acute inferior infarction (ED; 3/8/98).*

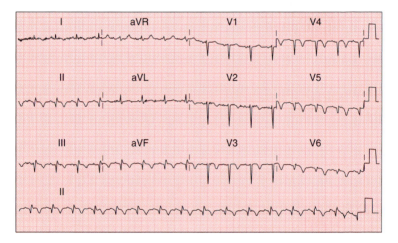

ECG 39: *Acute inferior and anterolateral infarction. Q waves and T wave inversions are seen in leads II, III, aVF, V4, V5 and V6 (Mr R; 26/1/98).*

True posterior infarction

True posterior infarction is rare. The dead window is situated posteriorly, therefore electrodes facing healthy tissues will record unopposed positive forces manifested by dominant R waves in leads V1 and V2 (Figure 17 and ECGs 40–41).

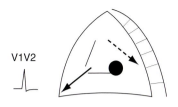

Figure 17: *True posterior infarction.* *Unopposed positive vectors are inscribed as dominant R waves in leads V1 and V2.*

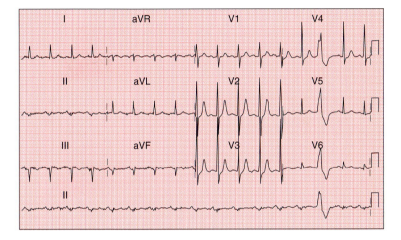

ECG 40: *Inferior and true posterior infarction. Q waves are seen in leads II, III and aVF. Dominant R waves are present in leads V1 and V2 (JF; 6/7/98).*

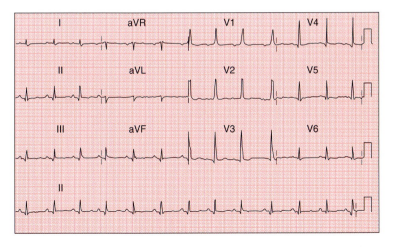

ECG 41: *True posterior infarction. Dominant R waves are present in leads V1 and V2. Probably significant, small Q waves are seen in the inferior leads (Mr R; 26/6/97).*

Progression of changes after Q wave infarction

The Q wave is nearly always permanent, although it can become less prominent over time. ST elevation, which is the first sign of infarction, resolves within a few hours: the T waves, on the other hand, revert to normal after several days or weeks (Figure 18).

In non Q wave (subendocardial) or partial thickness infarction, the ECG may revert to normal after days or weeks (Figure 19).

Examples of ECG changes in Q wave and non Q wave infarction are shown in ECGs 42–78, Figure 20, and ECGs 79–82.

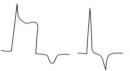

Acute   ST resolution   T resolution
(hours)   (days)

Figure 18: Progressive ECG changes after Q wave infarction.

No Q wave   Resolution to normal
(days or weeks)

Figure 19: Progression of non Q wave infarction.

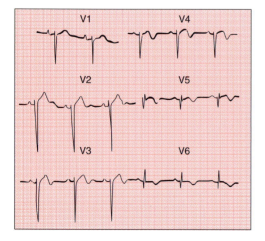

ECG 42: *Apical infarction. Q waves are visible in leads V5 and V6.*

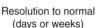

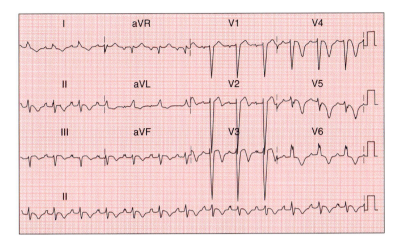

ECG 43: *This 87-year-old man had a subendocardial infarction in September 1996 (VS; 10/9/96).*

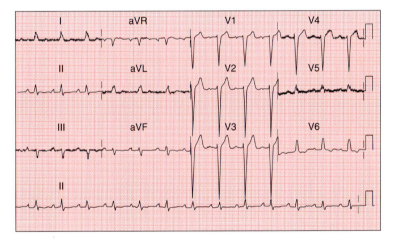

ECG 44: *He made a good recovery with medical treatment, as seen in this trace taken 7 months later (VS; 14/4/97).*

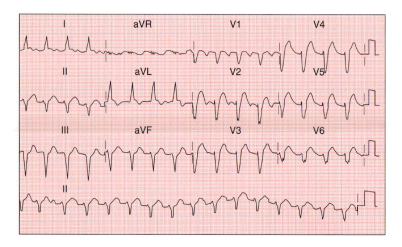

ECG 45: *A further 7 months later, the patient suffered anterior infarction with left bundle branch block. ST segment elevation is visible in the precordial leads with reduced R wave progression anterolaterally. The patient died. Subendocardial infarctions carry a bad prognosis (VS; 4/11/97).*

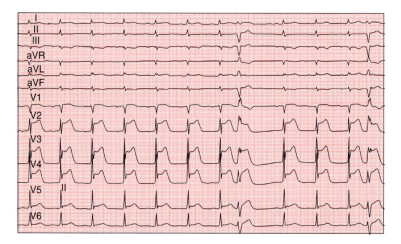

ECG 46: *Trace obtained during catheterisation of the left internal mammary artery in an elderly patient who had undergone bypass surgery several years previously. Marked anterior ischaemic changes are noted. The patient died soon after the procedure (CC; 23/4/98).*

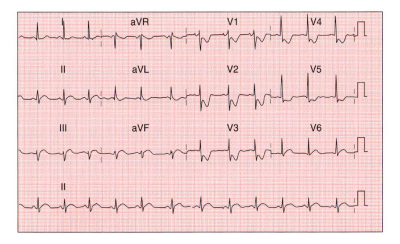

ECG 47: *Elderly female patient with subendocardial anterior infarction. Reciprocal ST segment elevation is visible in leads III and aVF. The patient died on the way to catheter laboratory five days after this event (HP; 11/7/99).*

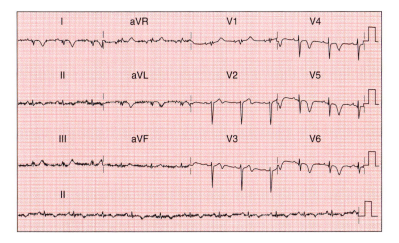

ECG 48: *Anterolateral infarction. Q waves are present in leads I and aVL. Reduced R waves are seen in leads V4, V5 and V6 and there are marked lateral T wave inversions (Mr E; 28/2/96).*

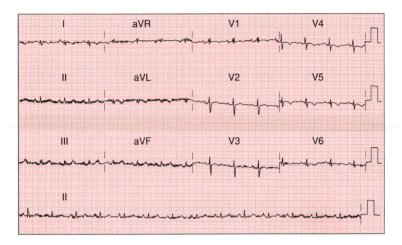

ECG 49: *The same patient 1 month after bypass surgery, showing marked improvement in ECG indices (Mr E; 10/5/96).*

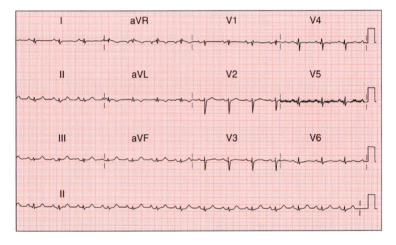

ECG 50: *A further 3 months later, there are minor residual Q waves in leads I and aVL with T wave inversion. Reduced R wave progression over leads V4–V6 is maintained (Mr E; 11/8/96).*

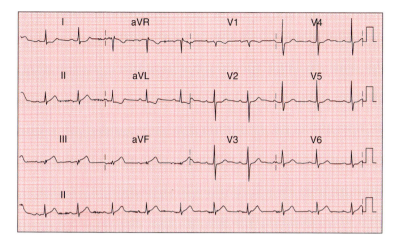

ECG 51: *Early changes of acute inferior infarction. ST segment elevation is present in leads III and aVF. Reciprocal changes are seen in leads I and aVL (FL; 15:10—28/4/96).*

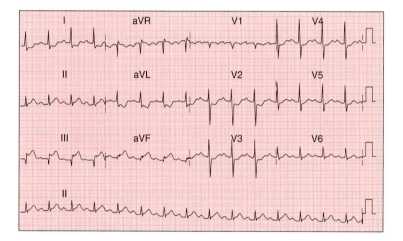

ECG 52: *Some four and a half hours later, Q waves are seen in leads III and aVF with ST elevation and reciprocal changes in I, aVL and V2–V5 (FL; 19:35—28/4/96).*

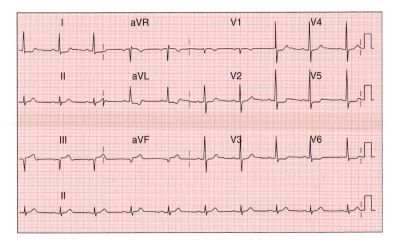

ECG 53: A further 24 hours later, inferior infarction is established. Q waves are visible in leads III and aVF, with minor ST segment elevation. There are resolving reciprocal changes (FL; 29/4/96).

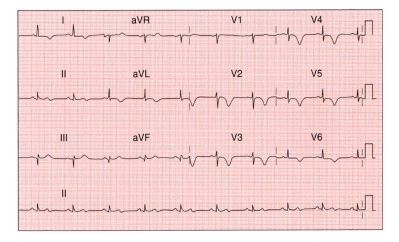

ECG 54: This 83-year-old female presented with subendocardial anterior infarction (BE; 5/5/96).

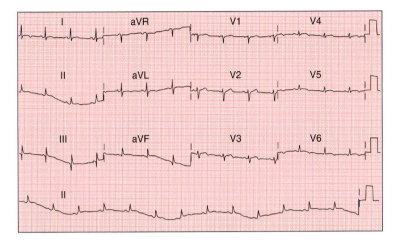

ECG 55: *There was marked improvement in ECG indices 10 days later, following bypass surgery (BE; 15/5/96).*

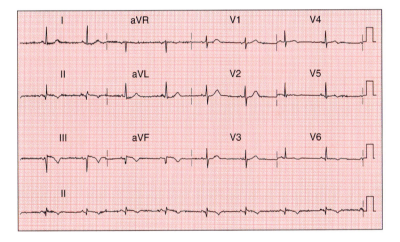

ECG 56: *Acute inferior infarction (HT; 28/11/96).*

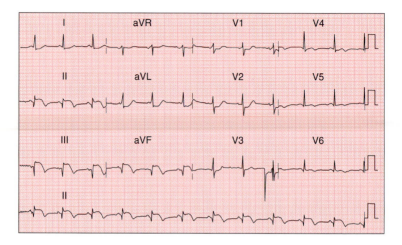

ECG 57: *ECG changes are worse 24 hours later. Reciprocal ST segment depressions are visible in leads V1 and V3 (HT; 29/11/96).*

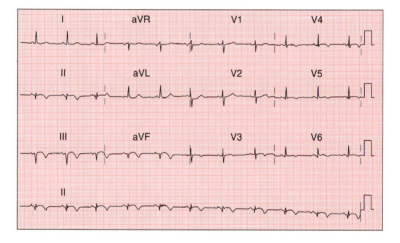

ECG 58: *One week later, after successful angioplasty of the right and left anterior descending coronary arteries. There is improvement in the inferior territory with minor T wave ischaemic changes in the LAD territory (HT; 6/12/96).*

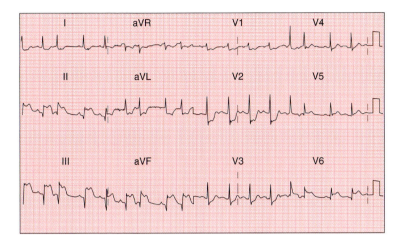

ECG 59: *The ECG of this 70-year-old male with acute inferior infarction showed widespread reciprocal ST depressions. The patient was given thrombolysins (RW; 6/10/95).*

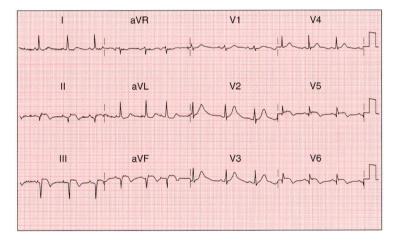

ECG 60: *After 2 days the reciprocal changes have largely disappeared. The inferior ST changes are resolving, but Q waves are evident (RW; 8/10/95).*

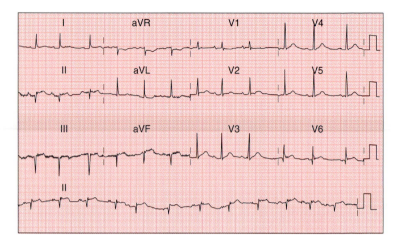

ECG 61: *After a further 3 days only the inferior Q waves remain in leads II, III and aVF (RW; 11/10/95).*

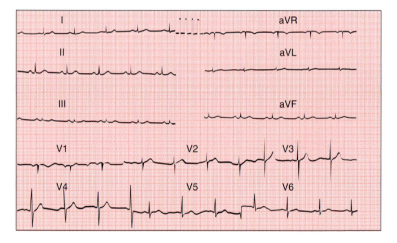

ECG 62: *This 52-year-old patient has a normal ECG (AS; 15/4/85).*

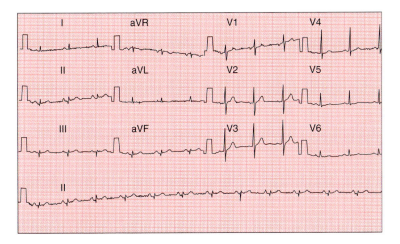

ECG 63: *Ten years later, there are Q waves indicating inferior infarction. The patient was unaware of this (silent myocardial infarction) (AS; 4/9/95).*

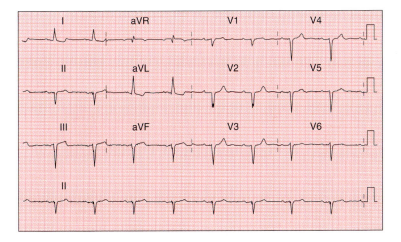

ECG 64: *ECG showing inferior and anterolateral Q waves with no R waves in leads V4–V6, indicating widespread infarcted territories (SK; 10/9/99).*

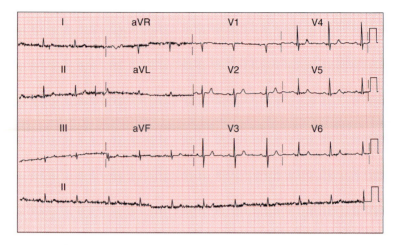

ECG 65: *Normal ECG in an elderly female patient in her mid-80s (HI; 1/3/99).*

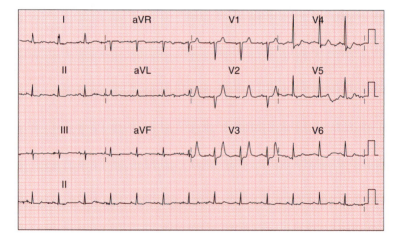

ECG 66: *The same patient presented with chest pain 4 months later. There are peaked T waves in leads V2 and V3 with some ST segment depressions in leads V3 and V4; cardiac enzyme levels were elevated (HI; 27/7/99).*

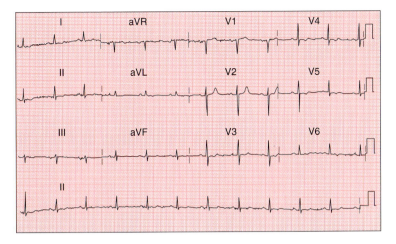

ECG 67: *ECG changes resolved, with only minor lateral T wave inversions remaining. At catheterisation, the patient was found to have three vessel disease, which was treated medically (HI; 6/9/99).*

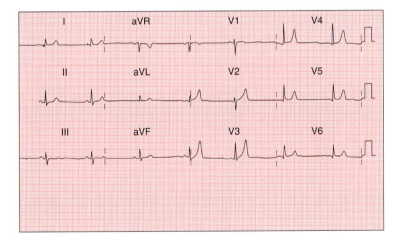

ECG 68: *This patient was due to have a mitral valve replacement and had a normal coronary arteriogram (PM; 31/5/99).*

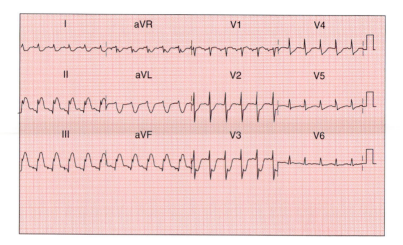

ECG 69: *The patient suffered a cardiac arrest in ITU after mitral valve replacement; there is acute inferior ST segment elevation with marked reciprocal changes in leads V2–V4. The patient was resuscitated successfully. The acute changes are due to coronary emboli, ?calcium, ?air (PM; 3/6/99).*

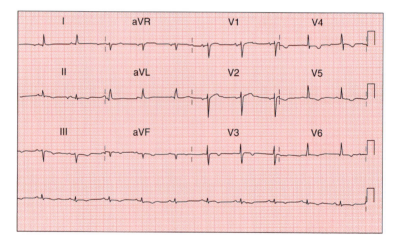

ECG 70: *Inferior Q waves with anterolateral T wave inversions are seen 1 week later (PM; 11/6/99).*

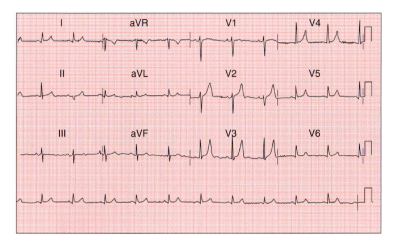

ECG 71: *All ECG indices returned to normal 4 months later (PM; October 1999).*

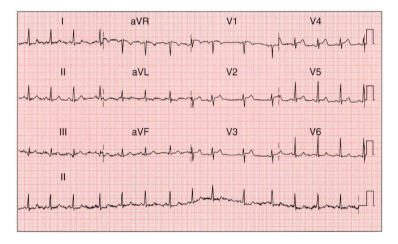

ECG 72: *This patient had angina at rest due to coronary arterial spasm. There are ST segment elevations in leads V2–V4 (Mr K; 1/1/89).*

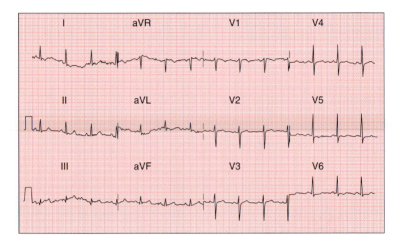

ECG 73: *Full resolution (Mr K; 26/4/99).*

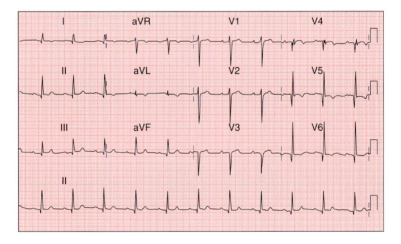

ECG 74: *Anteroapical infarction with deep Q waves in leads V3–V6 (RM; 30/11/98).*

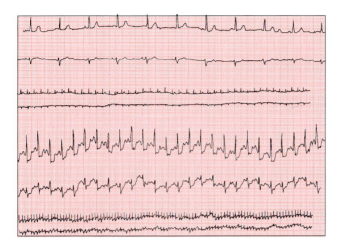

ECG 75: *24-hour Holter monitor showing acute ST segment depressions. The patient was unaware of her symptoms, in other words she had silent ischaemia (KB; 18/12/98).*

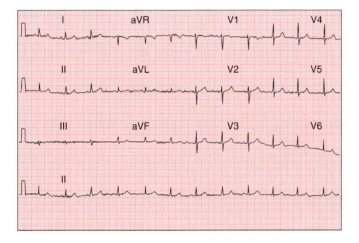

ECG 76: *This young Japanese patient has a normal electrocardiogram (CH; 24/12/94).*

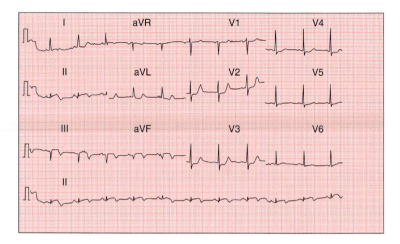

ECG 77: *5 months later the same patient presented with acute inferior infarction (CH; 13/5/95).*

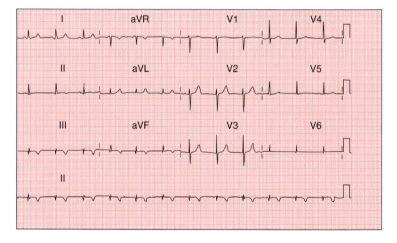

ECG 78: *Good resolution is evident 4 months later. Cardiac catheterisation revealed spontaneous dissection of a coronary artery (see Figure 20) (CH; 5/9/95).*

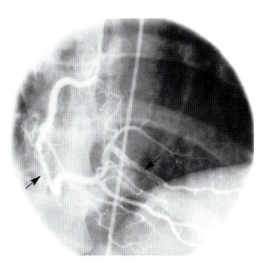

Figure 20: *Right coronary arteriogram from the same patient (ECG 78) showing dissection of the right coronary artery, which is well seen distally. The patient made a spontaneous recovery.*

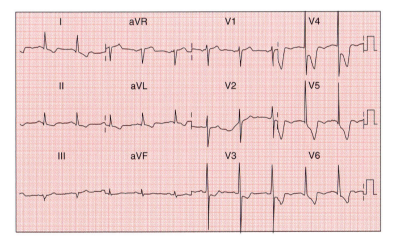

ECG 79: *Unstable angina with marked anterolateral ischaemic changes. Cardiac catheterisation showed critical mainstem stenosis. The patient underwent surgery on the same day (MK; 5/12/95).*

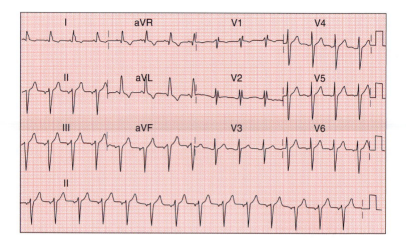

ECG 80: *The patient made a good recovery; 6 days after surgery, right bundle branch block is now evident (MK: 11/12/95).*

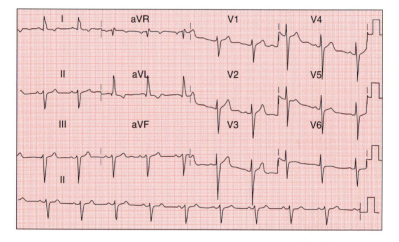

ECG 81: *After a further 3 years the patient is well, with some reduction of R wave progression (MK; 6/11/98).*

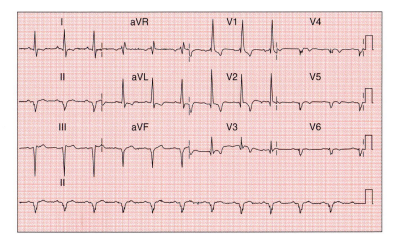

ECG 82: *Documented inferior and anterolateral infarctions with right bundle branch block. Q waves are seen in leads V2, V3, II, III and aVF (Mr J; 12/6/99).*

Further signs of ischaemic changes on ECG

- New, tall and peaked T waves may appear as a result of narrowing or obstruction of an epicardial artery; 'hyperpolarisation' occurs in the epicardial layer.
- Depression of the ST segment with T wave inversion in the lateral leads can be caused by acute elevation of left ventricular end diastolic pressure (related to subendocardial ischaemia).
- Distortion of the terminal QRS complex with reduced S waves can appear as a result of late depolarisation of the Purkinje system.
- Reduction of R wave progression over precordial leads indicates loss of LV musculature (also seen in obesity and emphysema).

Notes on Q wave

A Q wave is considered abnormal when it is:

- 0.03 secs (30 miliseconds) in duration, or greater than 25% of the following R wave;
- seen in leads normally showing an initial R wave.

Exercise ECG/stress test

Angina pectoris classically occurs during physical exertion. The oxygen demand of the myocardium exceeds the supply because of narrowing of the coronary arteries. This process eventually results in chest pain which is fairly characteristic. The pain radiates from the pericardium to the throat, and down the arms, and is relieved by interruption of the physical exertion or by inhaling, sucking or chewing nitroglycerine. Ischaemia can also manifest as breathlessness, caused by elevation of left ventricular end diastolic pressure. Silent ischaemia refers to evidence of myocardial ischaemia (ST changes) in the absence of pain. This is particularly evident in diabetics who suffer from autonomic nervous dysfunction.

Stress testing is performed by means of a standardised treadmill or bicycle (ergometry). The test should never be undertaken in a patient who has not been fully examined; it would be dangerous in the presence of congestive cardiac failure, rhythm abnormality or hypertension, or immediately after an infarct. It should be noted that certain drugs, such as digoxin, cause ST or T wave changes. Beta-blockers slow down the heart, preventing the heart rate response that is necessary to provoke an attack of angina. A supine ECG is required to ascertain that there are no acute changes before the stress test is undertaken. On standing, there may be certain ECG changes that are not necessarily abnormal, hence the need for a supine trace. Modern equipment provides heart rate, blood pressure and oximetry measurements with computer analysis of the ECG changes.

Both the treadmill and bicycle are standardised (according to the Bruce protocol) so that after 3 minutes of exercise the load is automatically increased until the patient is unable to proceed, or ECG abnormalities develop (for example ischaemia or arrhythmia), or there is a drop or rise in blood pressure beyond normal levels. The abnormality on the ECG that indicates an ischaemic response consists of a horizontal ST depression of at least 1 mm of 80 milliseconds duration (ECGs 83–86). The stress test should be abandoned at 4-5 mm depression of the ST wave.

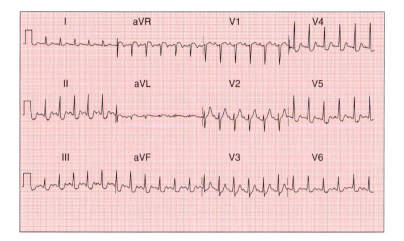

ECG 83: *Positive stress test in a patient with coronary artery disease. At a heart rate of 139 beats per minute, with symptoms of angina, the patient develops marked ST segment depressions in the inferior and lateral leads (II, III, aVF, V5 and V6) (LL; 11/11/96).*

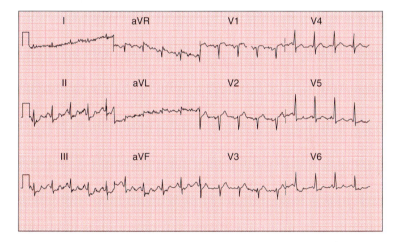

ECG 84: *Positive stress test with angina at a heart rate of only 107 beats per minute. ST segment depressions are seen in the inferior leads and in lead V6 (CW; 29/11/99).*

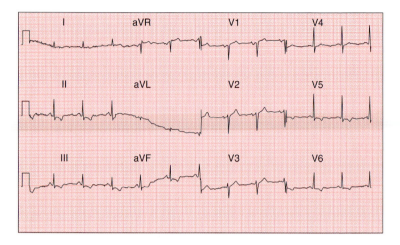

ECG 85: *During recovery at a heart rate of 71 beats per minute, classical T wave inversions occur in the same leads. These T wave inversions during recovery are pathognomonic for coronary artery disease. The patient had three vessel disease at coronary angiography (CW; 29/11/99).*

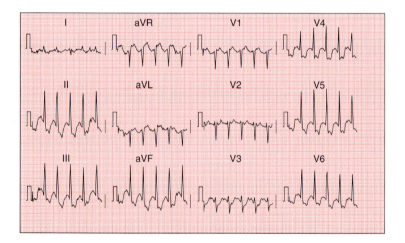

ECG 86: *Middle-aged female patient with severe aortic stenosis. Marked ST segment depressions during exercise at 158 beats per minute are noted in the inferior lateral leads. The coronary arteriogram was normal (AS; 3/7/91).*

Other ECG abnormalities on stress testing

ST elevation, rhythm or conduction disturbances can develop. A drop in blood pressure indicates severe coronary artery disease or a vasovagal response caused by hyperventilation with peripheral vasodilatation. In such instances, the patient is monitored in a horizontal position until recovered. Full resuscitative facilities must be available (defibrillator, cardiac drugs, oxygen and suction apparatus). The test is usually performed by technicians with a doctor in attendance. Complications are rare when the test is carried out properly and the personnel are well trained. However, occasional infarction can occur and fatalities are on record. The patient is observed for 5-10 minutes after the stress test, or longer if complications arise, with continuous ECG and blood pressure evaluation. The severity of a positive stress test—that is, the degree of—ischaemia is judged by the duration of the exercise, the appearance time of either symptoms or ECG changes, heart rate, blood pressure and oxygen saturation response. The latter reflects left ventricular and pulmonary function. Abnormal levels will occur with chronic pulmonary disease, right to left shunting or pulmonary oedema.

The occurrence of supraventricular and particularly ventricular arrhythmias (other than occasional extrasystoles), the appearance of bundle branch block or conduction defects, or a delayed decrease in heart rate during the first minute after the exercise are all parameters indicating a negative prognosis.

It has to be made quite clear that a positive stress test does not necessarily indicate underlying coronary pathology. ST and T wave changes during exercise can occur for other reasons:

- a false positive test (occurs in up to 5% of the population, more frequently in female patients [ECG 87]);
- related to hypertension;
- related to hyperventilation;
- associated with aortic valve disease (mainly severe aortic stenosis) or hypertrophic cardiomyopathy (ECG 86).

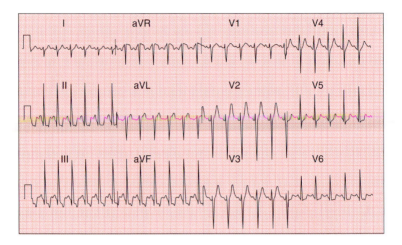

ECG 87: *This young patient, a professional diver, had a routine stress test that indicates coronary artery disease based on ST depressions with T wave inversions in the inferolateral lead (V6). The patient has no symptoms and coronary arteriography is entirely normal. This is an example of a false positive stress test (JB; 16/11/99).*

Nuclear (isotope) stress exercise testing (scintigraphy)

Intravenous radioactive substances (thallium, technetium) are injected during exercise supplemented by coronary vasodilators (dipyridamole or adenosine). Gamma camera pictures are obtained during exercise and subsequently at rest. Pictures of the isotope within the myocardium underline areas of underperfusion during exercise with improved flow after resting (indicating reversible ischaemic changes).

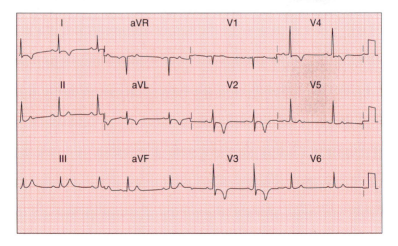

ECG 88: *This 86-year-old man presented with severe unstable angina. His cardiac enzyme levels were not elevated. He was treated medically (PR; 16/4/95).*

These findings relate to occlusive or stenotic lesions affecting the coronary arteries (ECGs 88, 89 and Figure 21).

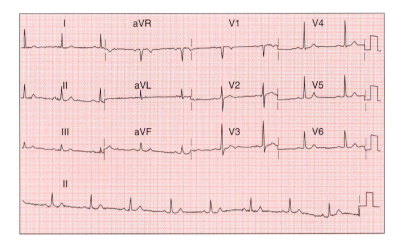

ECG 89: *After a strongly positive myocardial perfusion study (see Figure 21), the patient underwent stenting of a tight LAD lesion 3 days after admission. This produced a good result and total resolution of ECG changes (PR; 19/4/95).*

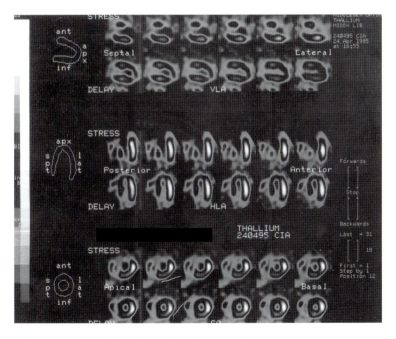

Figure 21: Myocardial perfusion stress test in three oblique views. *The upper pictures were taken during stress, and the bottom pictures after a period of recovery. In all views there is some resumption of flow in the LAD territory during recovery, indicating reversible ischaemic changes in the apex, anterior wall and septum. A tight LAD stenosis was confirmed at angiography (PR; April 1995).*

Stress echocardiography

This investigation involves echocardiographic imaging of the left ventricle at rest and during infusion with dobutamine and atropine. The purpose is to detect areas of undercontractile LV musculature related to regional coronary pathology (regional wall motion abnormality).

Angina at rest (variant or Prinzmetal angina)

Angina pain occurs at rest, rather than related to physical exertion. It can be brought on by mental stress or nightmares. The symptoms are similar to effort angina, and usually occur in advanced three vessel disease (LAD, circumflex and right coronary arteries) or mainstem disease. Less frequently, localised coronary arterial spasm can be demonstrated (ST elevation) or provoked (ergonovine test) during coronary angiography.

Management consists of calcium antagonists, potassium channel openers and nitrates (beta-blockers are contraindicated).

Unstable angina

In unstable angina the classical symptoms in a patient who was previously stable change so that the pain becomes more intense, occurs at rest, is provoked by less physical exertion and/or becomes less responsive to usual medication. Unstable angina is now considered a medical emergency requiring hospitalisation with aggressive management (medical and/or interventional). This consists of intravenous nitrates, heparin and/or clopidogrel, aspirin, usually followed by angiography which will indicate the need for percutaneous transluminal coronary angioplasty (PTCA) with or without stenting, or even coronary artery bypass surgery (CABG).

Other ischaemic heart diseases

Syndrome X

Syndrome X is characterised by exertional angina. Classical ST changes are observed during exercise stress testing, but coronary arteriography shows no obvious disease in the epicardial arteries. The pathology is believed to reside within the myocardial vessels, caused by either abnormal resistance to flow or some metabolic disorder.

Patients usually respond to beta-blockers, calcium antagonists, potassium channel openers, nitrates or a combination of any of these. Oestrogens appear to have a beneficial effect in some women.

Hibernating myocardium

Hibernating myocardium is a chronic state of muscle underperfusion. This results in reduced LV function, which usually responds to revascularisation—in other words, viable muscle is not functioning but is able to return to normal contractility after reperfusion.

Stunned myocardium

Stunned myocardium follows an acute event resulting from myocardial ischaemia that persists after coronary reperfusion. The situation usually remits and responds to inotropes.

Cardiogenic shock

Caused by a large infarct with hypotension, profuse sweating, vasoconstriction and pre-renal failure. The mortality can approach 70%. Early aggressive intervention is associated with a better six months prognosis.

Other ECG indices

Other ECG indices can be used to assess prognosis after myocardial infarction. These are listed below.

- Ventricular late potentials: low amplitude, high frequency electrical signals which are seen at the end of QRS complexes (using specialised equipment). These have been used to predict the development of arrhythmias after myocardial infarction. However, the predictive accuracy of the technique is low.
- Heart rate variability: used to obtain prognostic information after myocardial infarction by analysis of beat to beat variations of RR intervals. Vagal influence after myocardial infarction has a significant prognostic value.
- QT dispersion: measures differences between maximal and minimal QT intervals on a 12 lead ECG. Lengthening of the QT interval after myocardial infarction predicts the development of ventricular arrhythmias.

- Heart rate turbulence: found in low risk patients after MI by analysis of acceleration or deceleration after a single ventricular premature beat (VPB). A small risk of mortality has been found in patients who do not show this response.

Notes on ST changes

ST elevation
- Seen in normal subjects (in precordial leads)
- usual in black people (known as high uptake)
- ST elevation is otherwise a sign of:
  acute myocardial infarction
  acute coronary spasm (variant angina pectoris)
  left ventricular aneurysm
  pericardial effusion

ST depression
- always abnormal
- usually due to ischaemia
- seen in patients on digoxin
- associated with left ventricular hypertrophy (strain pattern)

Historical notes

RA Bruce (1916–) Professor of Medicine, Seattle, USA. Originator of 'Bruce protocol', laying down stress test guidelines.

M Prinzmetal (1908–) Professor of Cardiology, UCLA, California, USA. Described 'variant' angina due to coronary arterial spasm (1955).

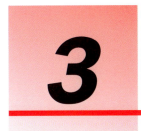

3 Conduction impairment

Sinus arrhythmia

Sinus arrhythmia is normal in children. It is abnormal in adults but not indicative of specific pathology. The heart accelerates during inspiration and slows during expiration (ECG 90).

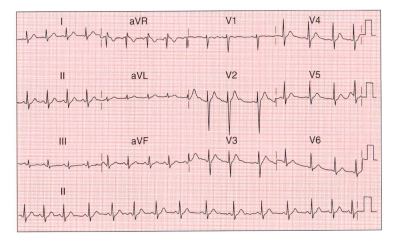

ECG 90: *Young medical student with sinus arrhythmia, seen at the bottom rhythm strip in lead II. Acceleration and deceleration of the heart are related to respiration. This is a normal finding in young adults; it is said to have pathological connotations later in life (MS; 28/5/99).*

Wandering pacemaker

Wandering pacemaker is seen usually with sinus arrhythmia, with the same clinical significance. The sinus pacemaker may move location within the SA node from beat to beat. This shows up as a change in P wave size and PR interval.

Sinus bradycardia

Sinus bradycardia is defined as a sinus rate below 50 beats per minute with otherwise normal conduction (ECG 91). It occurs mainly in patients taking beta-blockers but also occurs in hypothyroidism, obstructive jaundice and raised intracranial pressure. It is physiological in athletes and is seen in chronotropic incompetence—see next page for definitions.

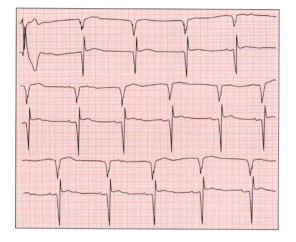

ECG 91: *A 90-year-old patient with marked sinus bradycardia and dizzy spells. 24-hour Holter ambulatory recording was performed on two channels, the lower ones showing the P waves more clearly. The upper strip shows a ventricular rate of 36 beats per minute, suggesting complete heart block. The last two complexes in the second strip confirm independent P waves (LC; 7/12/99).*

Sinus tachycardia

Sinus tachycardia is defined as a sinus rate over 100 beats per minute. It is normal in childhood. In adults it is a physiological response to exercise or a reaction to numerous insults such as fever, anaemia, hyperthyroidism, anxiety or heart failure. It can occur in response to certain drugs such as amlodipine, nifedipine, sympathomimetic agents, atropine, adrenaline, or isoprenaline.

Sinoatrial disease

Sinoatrial slowing can be physiological (for example in athletes) or acquired in response to old age (fibrosis), atheromatous disease or certain drugs (such as digoxin, beta-blockers and verapamil).

Definitions of sinoatrial disease are listed below.

- Sinoatrial block: a non-conducted P wave (not to be confused with an atrial premature beat arising in a refractory period).
- Sinoatrial arrest: a complete PQRST cycle is missing.
- Sinoatrial tachycardia (within the SA node): this can be caused by a localised re-entry circuit (rare).
- Chronotropic incompetence: represents the inability to increase the heart rate in response to exercise, caused by slowing down of the SA node. Seen in elderly individuals.
- Sick sinus syndrome: also known as tachy/brady syndrome. Sinoatrial disease characterised by episodes of intermittent bradycardia, atrial fibrillation, atrial flutter and supraventricular tachycardia.

Changes characteristic of sinoatrial disease are illustrated in ECGs 92-98.

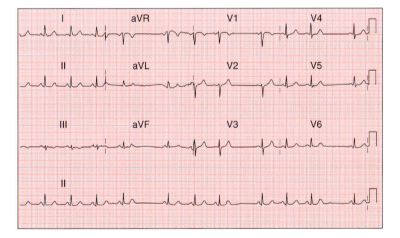

ECG 92: *A 48-year-old female patient with sinoatrial arrest. Rhythm strip lead II at the bottom shows complete absence of an entire PQRST complex (CM; 7/8/98).*

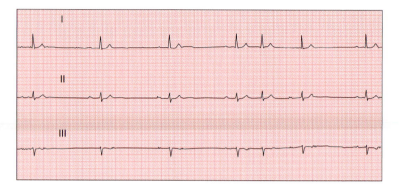

ECG 93: *A 57-year-old man with profound sinus bradycardia due to sinoatrial disease. The fifth complex is a junctional escape beat (Mr R; 3/4/97).*

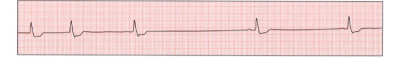

ECG 94: *This elderly woman developed profound sinus bradycardia after brainstem infarction (21/12/96).*

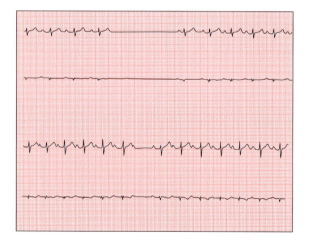

ECG 95: *A 33-year-old woman with sinoatrial disease. The upper strip shows sinus arrest. The bottom strip (in the middle) shows sinoatrial block (DL; 6/11/96).*

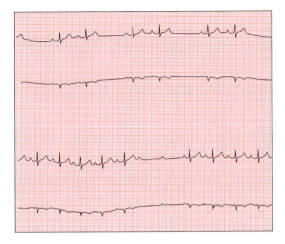

ECG 96: *The same patient. The upper strip shows sinoatrial arrest. The bottom strip shows a short spell of complete heart block. This is an unstable situation requiring permanent pacing (DL; 6/11/96).*

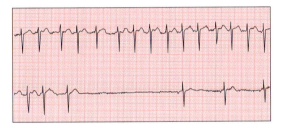

ECG 97: *Sinoatrial disease. Elderly patient with ischaemic heart disease. There is sinoatrial arrest with a long pause. This patient required a pacemaker. As a rule, pacing is indicated when pauses are more than 3 seconds in duration.*

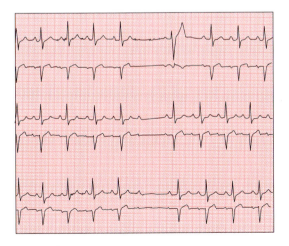

ECG 98: *Sinoatrial block. P waves are not conducted. The trace at the top shows sinoatrial arrest. The trace in the middle shows sinoatrial block (BB; 3/8/95).*

Atrioventricular block

First degree AV block

Prolonged PR interval over 0.2 seconds (20 ms), usually seen in the
elderly associated with coronary artery disease or acute rheumatic
carditis, or caused by certain drugs such as digoxin (ECGs 99–104).

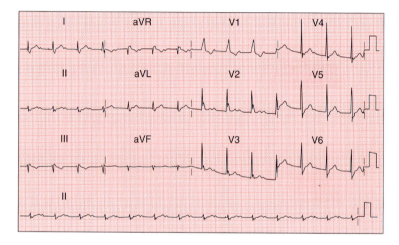

ECG 99: *This 80-year-old patient presented with dizzy spells. He had first degree heart block. There
is a prolonged PR interval, which can be seen clearly in leads V1 and V2. There is right bundle
branch block, left axis deviation, hence trifascicular block (MC; 19/2/95).*

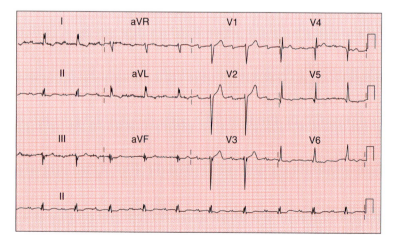

ECG 100: *Ischaemic heart disease. First degree heart block is indicated by the prolonged PR
interval (WN; 17/2/99).*

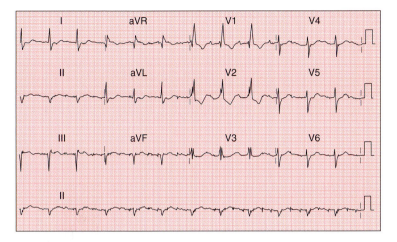

ECG 101: *This patient in his 80s has ischaemic heart disease. The ECG indicates first degree heart block. There is a right bundle branch block and left axis deviation (JK; 21/9/98).*

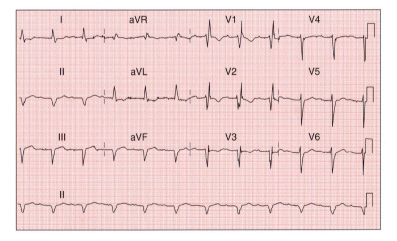

ECG 102: *Just over 1 year later, the first degree heart block is worsening (JK; 25/5/99).*

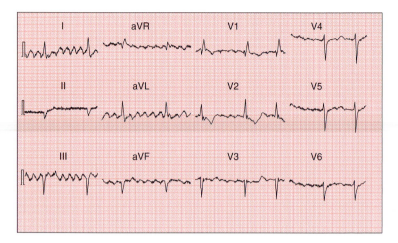

ECG 103: After a further 6 months, the patient went into atrial fibrillation (JK; 23/11/99).

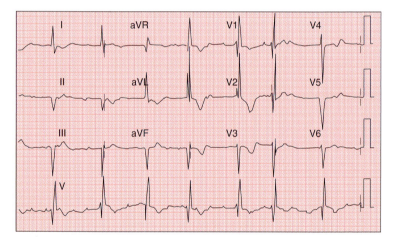

ECG 104: Five days later, there is complete heart block. The P waves are independent from the QRS complexes (JK; 28/11/99).

Second degree AV block

There are two types:

- **Mobitz I (Wenckebach):** the PR interval prolongs with each beat until an entire cycle is dropped (ECGs 105–106). It can occur in atheletes, the elderly and people with coronary artery disease. When associated with acute myocardial infarction, it may require temporary pacing.
- **Mobitz II:** regularly occurring non-conducted P waves (ECGs 107–108). The aetiology is the same as that of Mobitz I heart block.

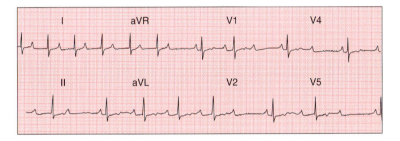

ECG 105: *Continuous strip showing episodic Wenckebach (Mobitz I) second degree heart block. The PR interval becomes prolonged in both strips and a ventricular complex is then dropped. The P wave is not conducted and the cycle restarts (Mr P; 29/3/97).*

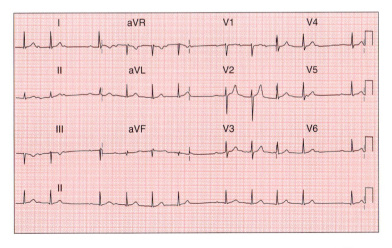

ECG 106: *A further example of Wenckebach phenomenon. The bottom strip (II) shows the PR interval to prolong. The complex is dropped due to a blocked P wave (DL; 3/2/97).*

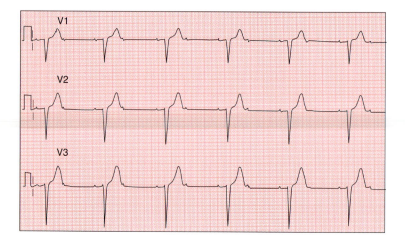

ECG 107: An 81-year-old lady with second degree heart block (Mobitz II). Each second P wave is not conducted (EL; 12/3/96).

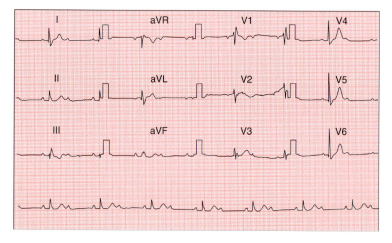

ECG 108: Another example of second degree heart block (Mobitz II) (HG; 4/5/95).

Third degree AV block

P waves discharge at their inherent rate, but cannot be conducted to the ventricles (an example of AV dissociation). If the QRS complexes are narrow (high grade AV block) the heart block is usually at the level of the bundle of His. The ventricular rate will be of the order of 50 beats per minute. If the QRS complexes are wide, the block is lower down and the rate will be between 30 and 40 beats per minute (ECGs 109-118). Adams–Stokes attacks refer to syncope caused by impaired cerebral circulation related to extreme bradycardia or ventricular arrest.

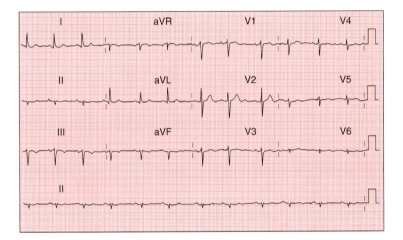

ECG 109: *This 70-year-old woman with ischaemic heart disease had normal sinus rhythm in July 1988 (QH; 28/7/98).*

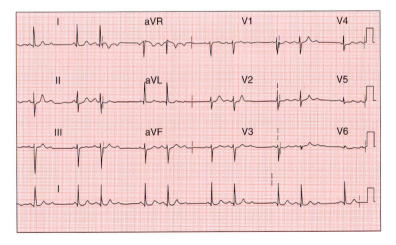

ECG 110: *Sinoatrial block was evident 1 month later (QH; 5/8/98).*

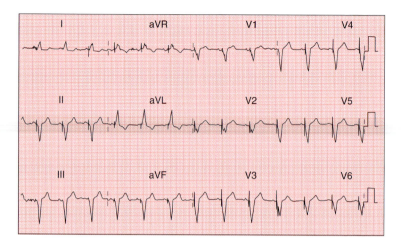

ECG 111: *The heart was pacing adequately (VDD). Two days later the AV sequential contraction is maintained through a single path lead. The electrode 'floating' in the right atrium senses the atrial P wave and sends a signal to the right ventricle, which is then paced (QH; 7/8/98).*

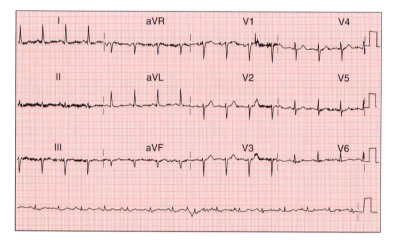

ECG 112: *Normal sinus rhythm (WP; 23/7/93).*

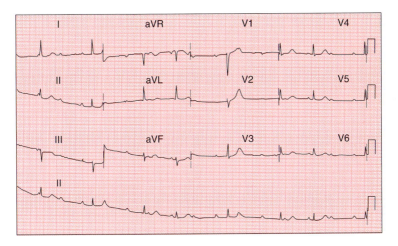

ECG 113: *The same patient, 5 years later, has complete heart block. The bottom strip (lead 2) shows P waves appearing at a normal rate. These are not conducted to the ventricles, which are beating independently at a rate of 40 beats per minute (WP; 26/11/98).*

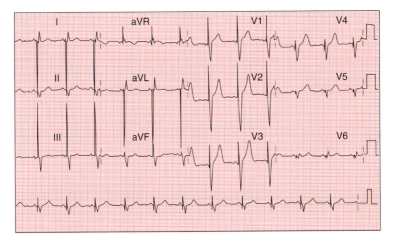

ECG 114: *The same patient with AV sequential pacing. Each P wave is followed by a paced signal (WP; 27/11/98).*

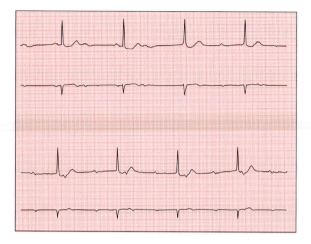

ECG 115: *Complete heart block on 24-hour Holter monitor. The ventricular heart rate is 34 beats per minute. The atria are beating independently at a faster rate (SW; 11/7/96).*

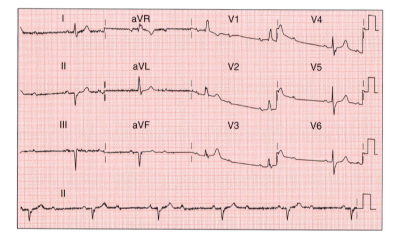

ECG 116: *This elderly man presented with second degree (Mobitz II) heart block (SJ; 8/5/95).*

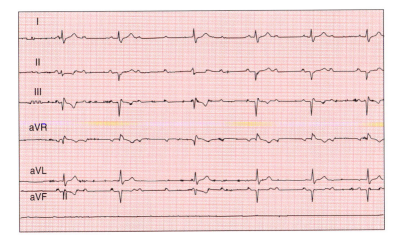

ECG 117: *The condition proceeded to complete heart block (SJ; 8/5/95).*

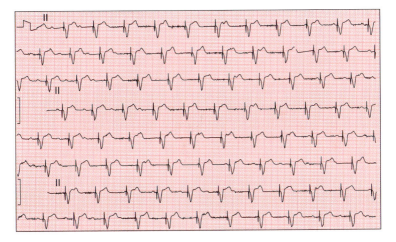

ECG 118: *VVI pacing in the same patient. The right ventricle is paced independently of P wave activity, which is seen to be unrelated to the pacing signals (SJ; 15/5/95).*

Management

- Atropine is of no use.
- Give isoprenaline by mouth or intravenous infusion.
- A temporary pacemaker can be useful, particularly after acute myocardial infarction.
- A permanent pacemaker may be necessary (see Chapter 8).
- Use an external pacemaker when other methods are unavailable.

Predisposing conditions

Conditions that predispose to third degree AV block include acute MI, calcified aortic valve disease, bifascicular and trifascicular block, cardiac surgery and occasionally drugs (beta-blockers and cocaine).

Congenital complete heart block

Congenital complete heart block is usually seen in children. The ventricular rate is around 60 beats per minute. Syncopal attacks are rare, but they do occur and permanent pacing may be required.

Bundle branch block

Normal conduction

Having reached the bundle of His, situated in the upper portion of the interventricular septum (IVS), the electrical impulse is transmitted to the bundles, supplying the right and left ventricles (right and left bundles). The right bundle is single and the left divides into two: the superior or anterior branch, and the inferior or posterior branch (Figure 22).

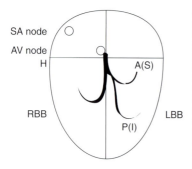

Figure 22: Conduction system. *The sinoatrial node discharges at an inherent rate of around 70 beats per minute in adults (faster in children). It is influenced by neurogenic and hormonal input. The impulse is 'filtered' down the AV node, enters the bundle of His and then travels to both right and left bundle branches. The left divides into an anterior (superior) and inferior (posterior) branch and thence ramifies through the Purkinje system to all parts of the ventricles (from endocardium to epicardium). SA node = sinoatrial node; AV node = atrioventricular node; H = His; RBB = right bundle branch; LBB = left bundle branch; A = anterior (S = superior); P = posterior (I = inferior).*

Right bundle branch block

Right bundle branch block (RBBB) occurs when there is an interruption of the right bundle below the bundle of His. The right ventricle is now electrically stimulated from the left ventricle (Figure 23).

In complete RBBB the QRS complex measures more than 0.10 seconds (100 ms). In partial or incomplete RBBB the QRS complex duration is less than 0.10 seconds (100 ms). 'M' shaped complexes are seen in leads V1–V2.

Right bundle branch block can be congenital and of no clinical importance. If acquired it bears a different connotation, indicating right ventricular pathology (ischaemia, pulmonary hypertension, pulmonary embolism, or congenital conditions such as ASD).

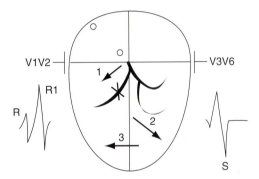

Figure 23: Right bundle branch block. *Vector 1 represents septal activation from left to right giving rise to a positive deflection in leads facing the right ventricle (R wave). Vector 2 represents left ventricular activation, that is, a negative wave (S wave) and Vector 3 represents late right ventricular activation (R1). These occur in electrodes facing the right ventricle. By contrast, left ventricular facing leads (I, aVL, V5, V6) will demonstrate a late negative S wave reflecting the delayed right ventricular depolarisation. Complete right bundle branch block refers to a QRS complex wider than 0.10 seconds (10 ms). Incomplete right bundle branch block occurs as above, but the QRS complex is less than 0.10 seconds (10 ms) in duration.*

Left bundle branch block

Left bundle branch block (LBBB) occurs when there is interruption of the left bundle below the bundle of His, affecting both anterior and inferior divisions.

In left bundle branch block the QRS complex duration is usually over 1.2 seconds (120 milliseconds). Left bundle branch block generally

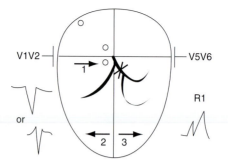

Figure 24: Left bundle branch block. *Septal activation originates from the right bundle (1) showing up an initial positive deflection in left ventricular facing leads. Right ventricular activation (2) is directed away, hence a negative S wave is produced. Vector 3 is caused by delayed LV depolarisation and is positive (RSR¹). In right ventricular facing leads it is usual to see a deep negative (Q) wave reflecting septal and late LV activity. Occasionally, if the right ventricle is activated earlier than the septum, a small positive R wave is seen.*

indicates left ventricular disease (such as hypertension, ischaemia, or valvar disease). Rarely, it can be congenital. 'M' shaped complexes are seen in leads V5-V6 (Figure 24).

In both right and left bundle branch block the ST/T wave pattern is inscribed in the opposite direction from the main QRS vectors. They do not indicate an underlying pathology.

Stress testing can be undertaken in patients with right bundle branch block. With left bundle branch block the ECG is not interpretable. Right bundle branch block with myocardial infarction will show an initial negative (Q) wave. Left bundle branch block with myocardial infarction is generally undiagnosable, although expertise may detect minor relevant abnormalities.

Hemiblocks

Anterior hemiblock

In anterior hemiblock there is interruption of the superior left bundle characterised by **left axis deviation**, the electrical impulse stimulating the left ventricle from below (Figure 25).

Inferior hemiblock

Inferior hemiblock shows up as **right axis deviation**, the impulse travelling downwards from the unaffected superior left bundle (Figure 26).

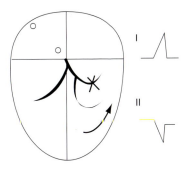

Figure 25: Left anterior hemiblock. *The upper portion of the left ventricle is stimulated from below, that is from the intact inferior bundle.*

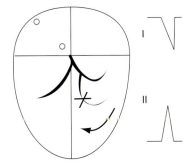

Figure 26: Inferior hemiblock. *The inferior bundle does not conduct. The signal travels downwards from the intact anterior bundle.*

Bifascicular block

Bifascicular block is right bundle branch block with either left or right axis deviation, or complete left bundle branch block. The former reflects interruptions through the right bundle on the one hand and the superior or inferior left bundle on the other. Complete left bundle branch block infers interruption of both superior and inferior bundles. Progression to complete heart block is feasible, particularly in an acute situation such as myocardial infarction, necessitating pacing.

Trifascicular block

Trifascicular block is the same as bifascicular block with additional prolongation of the PR interval (first degree AV block). Again, this can progress to complete heart block. These patients need careful supervision and are requested to report back in the event of dizzy spells or syncope. Examples from patients with bundle branch blocks are illustrated in ECGs 119-148.

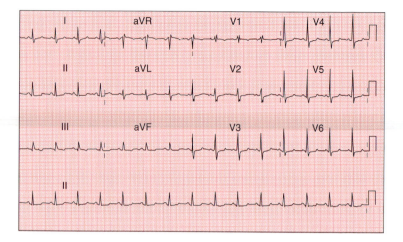

ECG 119: Incomplete right bundle branch block (Mr A; 20/6/97).

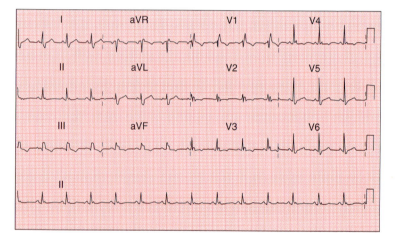

ECG 120: Complete right bundle branch block develops 12 months later. The QRS complex is now more prolonged. There is a deeper, wider S wave in leads I, V5 and V6 (Mr A; 8/6/98).

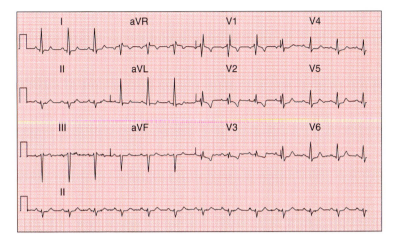

ECG 121: *Right bundle branch block with left axis deviation, constituting a bifascicular block (ML; 19/3/99).*

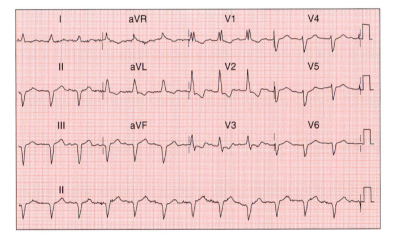

ECG 122: *Right bundle branch block with left axis deviation. There is a prolonged PR interval, constituting a trifascicular block. The patient developed subsequent complete heart block requiring permanent pacing (LC; 23/11/99).*

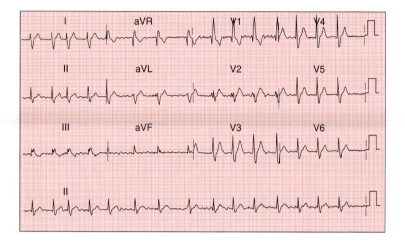

ECG 123: *Atrial fibrillation, right bundle branch block and right axis deviation, constituting a bifascicular block (SR; 12/11/99).*

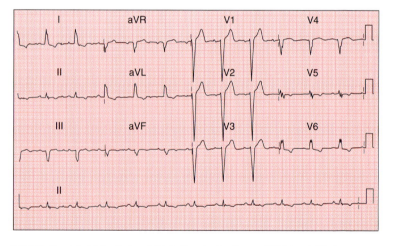

ECG 124: *Complete left bundle branch block. Normal axis with normal PR interval. This is a bifascicular block since both left bundles are blocked.*

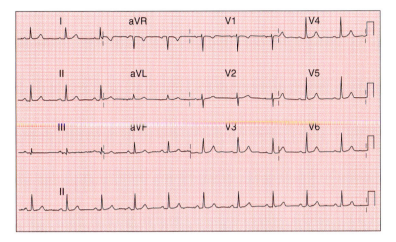

ECG 125: Normal conduction in a middle-aged woman with mild aortic stenosis (ST; 27/8/97).

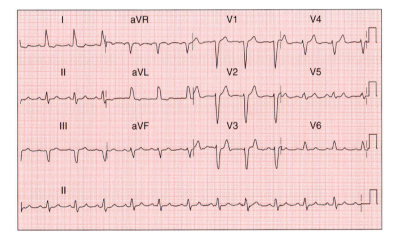

ECG 126: Left bundle branch block is seen in the same patient 2 years and 3 months later. There is a normal axis and normal PR interval with no worsening of the aortic valve gradient. There is no evidence of ischaemic heart disease, indicating progressive AV conduction dysfunction (ST; 30/11/99).

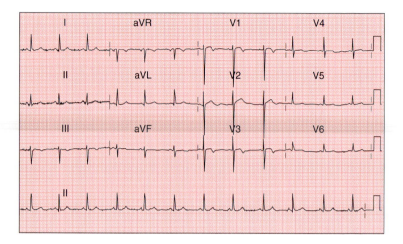

ECG 127: *This elderly woman with marked aortic stenosis has a fairly normal electrocardiogram, with T wave inversions in lead V3 (JS; 3/6/96).*

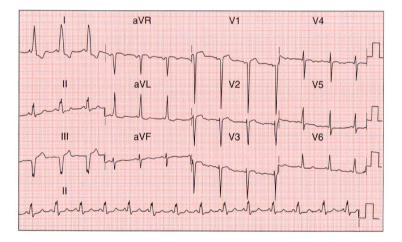

ECG 128: *Just over 2 years later showing complete left bundle branch block and left ventricular voltages. The patient underwent successful aortic valve replacement (JS; 10/7/98).*

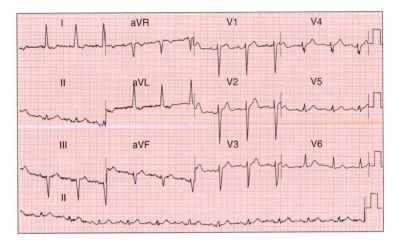

ECG 129: *ECG from an elderly woman with incomplete left bundle branch block (SR; 2/6/92).*

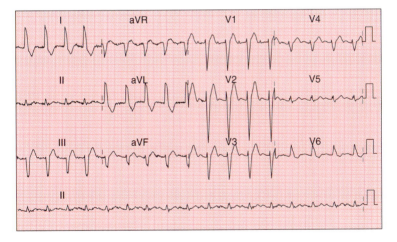

ECG 130: *After 7 years, the patient has progressed to complete left bundle branch block with first degree heart block. Normal axis maintained. This is a trifascicular block (SR; 12/1/99).*

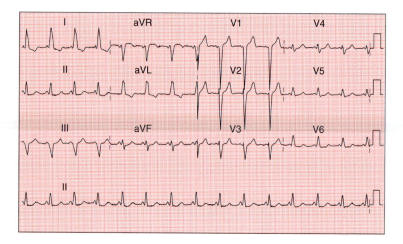

ECG 131: *The patient is an elderly woman, diagnosed with acute viral myocarditis. There is left ventricular failure and left bundle branch block (FO; 8/4/97).*

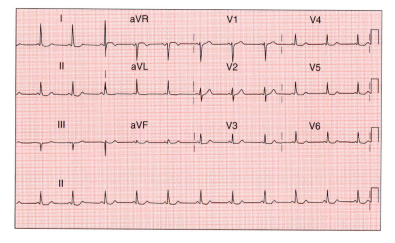

ECG 132: *The patient made a full recovery several months later. The ECG shows normal conduction, maintaining a short PR interval (FO; 9/7/97).*

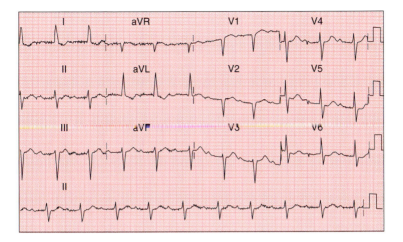

ECG 133: *ECG from a 77-year-old patient with ischaemic heart disease. There is an interventricular conduction defect (widened QRS complexes) and a left bundle branch block pattern. Left axis deviation and prolonged PR interval are best seen in the rhythm strip at the bottom (MB; 3/6/98).*

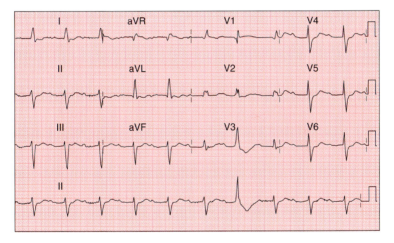

ECG 134: *Fifteen months later there is a prolonged PR interval and left axis deviation. The patient has developed right bundle branch block with clearly visible R1 waves in leads V1 and V2 and an S wave in lead I. This is an unusual situation and there is obviously still some conduction from the sinus node to the ventricles. The patient complained of dizzy spells (MB; 30/9/99).*

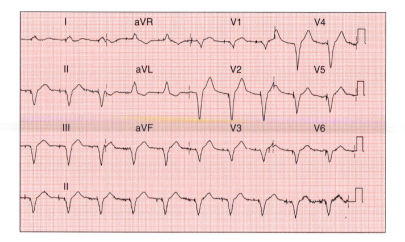

ECG 135: *The same patient following pacemaker implantation (DDD) (MB; 1/10/99).*

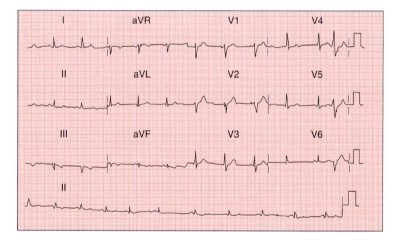

ECG 136: *Pre-bypass surgery ECG (SB; 4/2/87).*

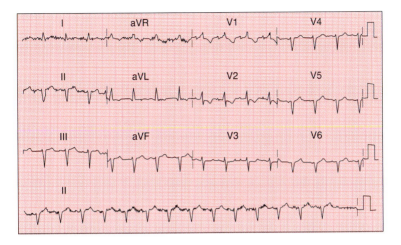

ECG 137: *Postoperative changes showing prolongation of the PR interval, right bundle branch block and left axis deviation. This is an example of surgical trauma to the conducting system (SB; 20/2/87).*

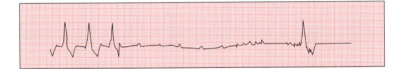

ECG 138: *The same patient developed ventricular asystole with only P waves visible. A pacemaker was implanted successfully (SB).*

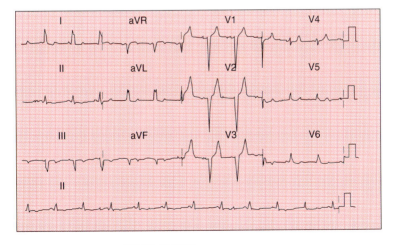

ECG 139: *Pre-bypass surgery ECG (AR; 26/3/86).*

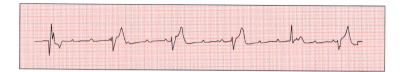

ECG 140: *The same patient developed complete heart block as a result of surgical trauma to the conducting system (AR; 29/3/86).*

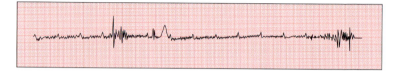

ECG 141: *Ventricular asystole. Only P waves are visible. This patient survived pacemaker implantation (AR; 4/4/86).*

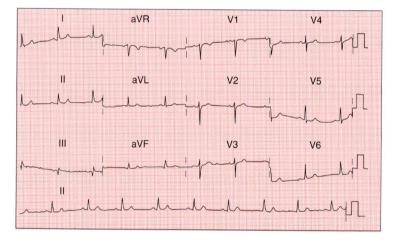

ECG 142: *Pre-operative (CABG) ECG, which is quite normal (FC; 20/11/87).*

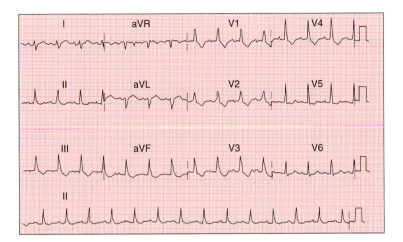

ECG 143: *Postoperative ECG showing right bundle branch block. There is a prolonged PR interval with right axis deviation, caused by surgical trauma to the conducting system (FC; 26/11/87).*

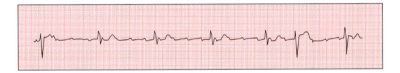

ECG 144: *The patient's condition progressed to complete heart block, which was treated by pacemaker insertion (FC; 30/11/87).*

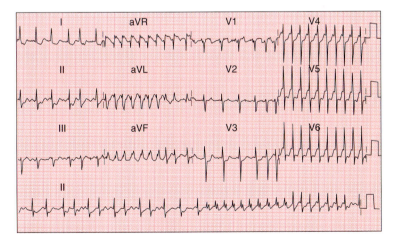

ECG 145: *ECG from an elderly woman with supraventricular arrhythmia showing marked ST depressions in the lateral leads with rate related bundle branch block developing towards the end of the rhythm strip (lead II) at bottom of the ECG. She was treated medically (Mrs L; 6/5/93).*

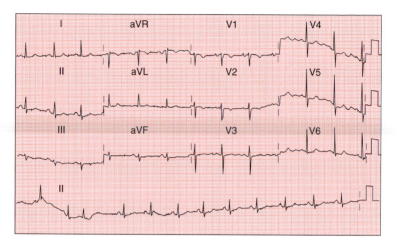

ECG 146: *The following day, the same patient had fully recovered. The bundle branch block is rate dependent due to 'fatiguing' of a bundle. Subsequent coronary arteriography was quite normal. The ischaemic changes reflect underperfusion caused by an increased heart rate with otherwise normal coronary arteries (Mrs L; 7/5/93).*

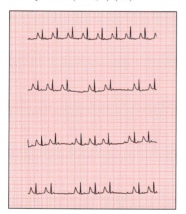

ECG 147: *Holter monitoring indicating sinoatrial block in a young, active 'sporty' female who complained of palpitation. This ECG appearance is often seen in healthy young adults. No medication is indicated and the prognosis is favourable (Ms G; 23/12/97).*

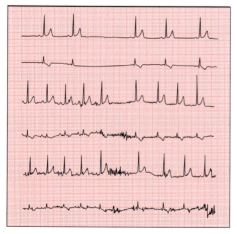

ECG 148: *Prolonged pause (2.53 seconds) caused by sinoatrial arrest in a young, athletic solicitor. As with the previous case, no medication is indicated and the prognosis is good (AB; 3/11/99).*

Carotid sinus syndrome

Following the application of pressure a hypersensitive carotid body can cause profound vagal activation resulting in extreme cases in ventricular asystole. Normal carotid massage causes sinus bradycardia. The manoeuvre is useful, occasionally, to terminate supraventricular arrhythmias, to bring in pacing activity when an increased heart rate inhibits the pacemaker setting and to slow down an atrial flutter, allowing the flutter waves to be recognised more easily (ECGs 149–152).

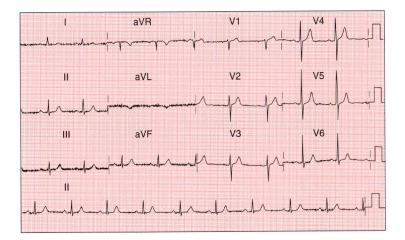

ECG 149: *Normal ECG from an elderly man with syncopal attacks attributed to cervical spondylosis (BH; 21/6/93).*

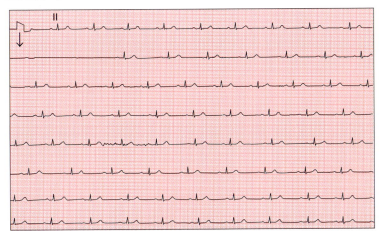

ECG 150: *Right carotid massage caused ventricular asystole. The patient had no further symptoms after pacemaker implantation. ↓ indicates right carotid massage (BH).*

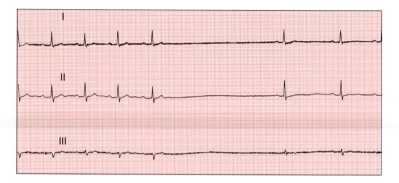

ECG 151: *ECG from a patient who presented with a CVA, with previous myocardial infarction. Right carotid massage caused profound bradycardia. The patient refused a pacemaker (2/3/99).*

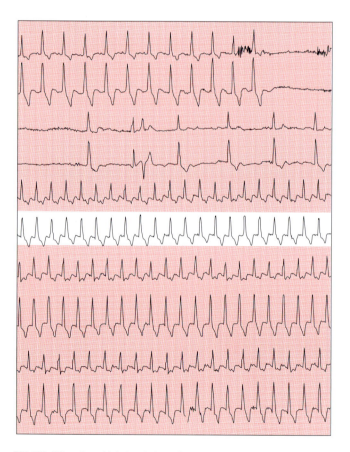

ECG 152: *This patient with ischaemic heart disease and bypass surgery reported numerous syncopal attacks. Repeated Holter monitoring was negative. On this occasion the patient was carrying a Holter when he had an argument with a taxi driver and collapsed. The top of the strip, which is continuous, shows the sinus tachycardia associated with aggravation, prolonged pause (cardiac arrest), slow recovery and the subsequent accelerated rhythm (Mr L; July 1994).*

Pre-excitation conduction: accessory pathways

Wolff–Parkinson–White (WPW) syndrome

This is an important ECG pattern to recognise as it mimics a number of different conditions. An accessory (congenital) bundle of Kent allows conduction from the atria to the ventricle resulting in early excitation (no AV nodal delay) of parts of the right or left ventricles (pre-excitation). The impulse travels down both the normal and abnormal pathways but moves at a faster rate down the latter. This pre-excitation results in a short PR interval. Having reached the ventricle through this abnormal pathway, the impulse has to travel through the myocardium as opposed to the normal conducting system. This slowed down impulse gives rise to a slurred delta wave on ECG. WPW syndrome can occur intermittently. It can be associated with rapid supraventricular arrhythmias (re-entry), atrial fibrillation or atrial flutter (no protection from AV nodal delay). The mechanism consists of a re-entry circuit, with the impulse moving down the normal pathway and re-entering the atria via the abnormal accessory pathway. Very fast supraventricular rates can ensue and rarely call progress to ventricular tachycardia and even ventricular fibrillation (ECGs 153–165).

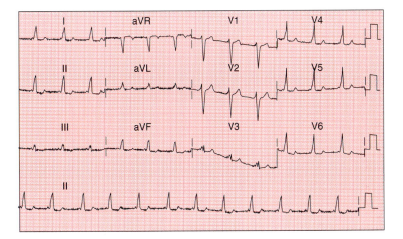

ECG 153: *Wolff–Parkinson–White syndrome, with a characteristic very short PR interval. Delta waves are best seen in leads V4–V6 (with slurring on upstroke of the R wave) (SR; 26/10/95).*

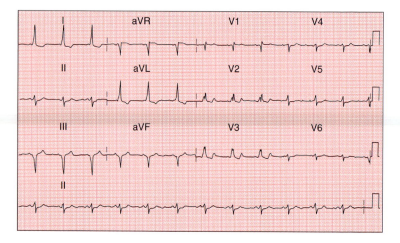

ECG 154: *WPW syndrome. There is a short PR interval, with delta waves in leads I and aVL. Note inferior Q waves (PN; 15/2/96).*

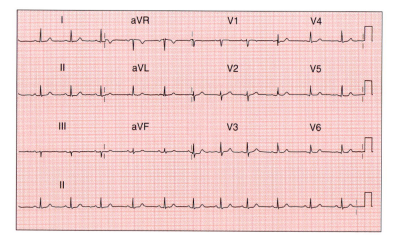

ECG 155: *The same patient, 2 years later after successful ablation. There is a normal PR interval with no delta or inferior Q waves. WPW can mimic infarction patterns (PN; 17/12/98).*

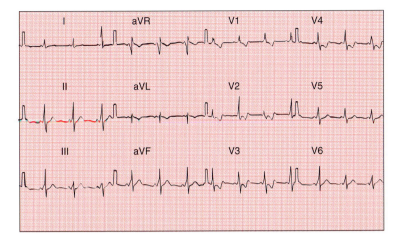

ECG 156: *ECG from a young man, showing classical WPW syndrome changes. There is a short PR interval and delta waves are well seen. In addition, there are abnormal T waves, which could be misconstrued as a sign of an ischaemic process (MS; 22/4/91).*

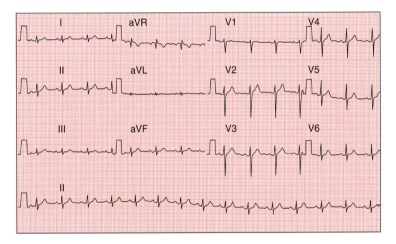

ECG 157: *After ablation of the accessory pathway, normality is restored (MS; 19/2/96).*

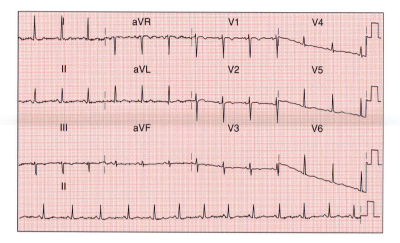

ECG 158: Fairly normal ECG from a middle-aged woman. The precordial T wave inversions are of no significance (FJ; 16/2/95).

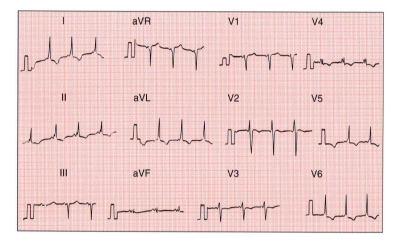

ECG 159: One month later, the ECG indicates classical WPW syndrome (FJ; 8/3/95).

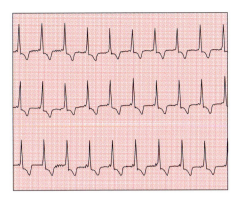

ECG 160: *The diagnosis is confirmed on Holter monitor. There is a short PR interval, with delta waves (FJ; 15/3/95).*

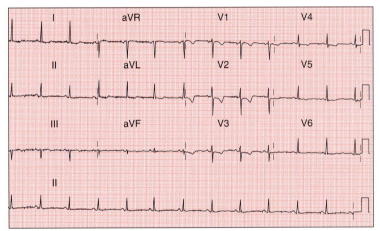

ECG 161: *After a further 4 years, there is normal conduction with marked anteroseptal T wave inversions. This an example of intermittent WPW syndrome (FJ; 5/7/99).*

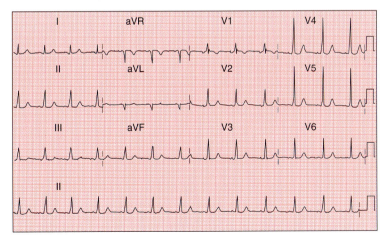

ECG 162: *WPW syndrome. Delta waves are apparent in leads II, III, aVF and V1. The PR interval is not particularly short (LK; 13/10/95).*

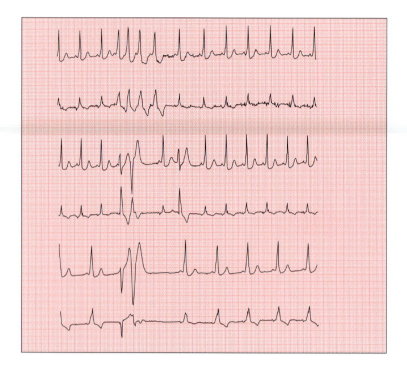

ECG 163: *24-hour Holter monitoring showing runs of supraventricular tachycadia in the same patient. This appearance could suggest a ventricular tachycardia (LK; 13/10/95).*

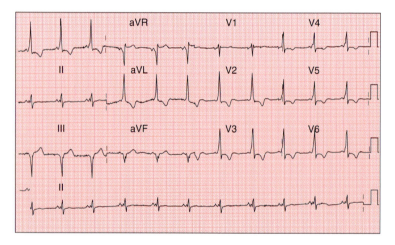

ECG 164: *Classical WPW changes in a 26-year-old woman. Note inferior Q waves and widespread T wave inversions (JD; 11/7/93).*

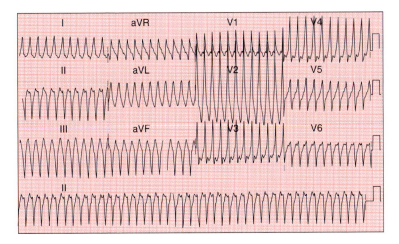

ECG 165: *ECG from the same patient showing a very fast supraventricular re-entry tachycardia. This could be confused with a ventricular tachycardia. Small retrograde P waves are discernible in lead I (JD; 25/7/93).*

Lown–Ganong–Levine syndrome

The typical ECG has a short PR interval (under 0.10 seconds [100 ms]) without a delta wave. The presence of an accessory pathway can promote rapid re-entry supraventricular tachycardias. The accessory pathway ends distally within the AV node or the bundle of His. The impulse does not stimulate the myocardium (unlike WPW syndrome) and hence no delta waves are seen (ECG 166).

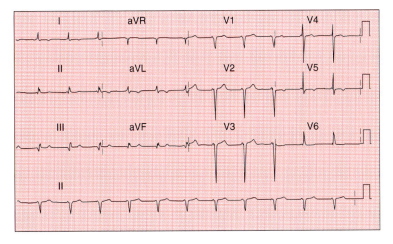

ECG 166: *Lown-Ganong-Levine syndrome. The short PR interval is clearly seen in lead VI. There are no delta waves. (KB-G; 23/11/95).*

Long QT interval

This ECG sign is associated with syncope caused by ventricular tachy-cardia. It can cause sudden death. Two separate syndromes are recognised: Jervel-Lange-Nielsen syndrome, which is associated with deafness and Romano Ward, which is familial and affects children.

Certain drugs prolong the QT interval. This can lead to ventricular arrhythmias (torsade de pointes), eg: quinidine, disopyramide, procainamide, sotalol, amiodarone and propafenone. Certain psychotropic drugs (phenothiazine, tricyclic antidepressants, lithium, and droperidol) and antihistamines (terfenadine) are known to prolong the QT interval and may cause sudden death.

Historical notes

AFS Kent (1863–1958) Professor of Physiology, Bristol University, Bristol, UK. Demonstrated muscular bridges between atria and ventricles.

L Wolff (1898–1972) American cardiologist, Massachusetts General Hospital, USA.

J Parkinson (1885–1976) English cardiologist, London Hospital, UK.

PD White (1886–1973) American cardiologist, Massachusetts General Hospital, USA. The Wolff-Parkinson-White syndrome was first published in 1930.

B Lown (born 1921) American cardiologist, Peter Brent, Brigham Hospital, Boston, USA. Nobel Peace Prize 1985.

WF Ganong (born 1924) American.

SA Levine (1891–1966) American cardiologist.

Lown-Ganong-Levine syndrome: short PR interval associated with supraventricular arrhythmias.

A Jervel (1901–1987) Professor of Medicine, Alleval Hospital, Oslo.

F Lange Nielsen. Contemporary of A Jervel.

Jervel-Lange-Nielsen syndrome: Prolonged QT interval associated with sudden death.

C Romano (born 1924) Professor of Paediatrics, Genoa, Italy.

OC Ward (born 1923) Professor of Clinical Paediatrics, Dublin, Ireland. Romano-Ward syndrome: Prolonged QT interval.

KF Wenckebach (1864–1940) Dutch cardiologist, Groningen and Vienna, Austria. Described periodically dropped beats (1899).

W Mobitz, Germany. Published work on partial conductor block.

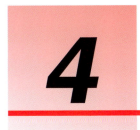

4

Rhythm disturbances

Arrhythmias are rhythms of the heart arising outside the normal conductive pathways or within them, but at an abnormal rate and with an abnormal ECG pattern. They are conventionally divided into two categories:

1) supraventricular arrhythmias, which originate from the atria or the AV node complex (junctional);
2) ventricular arrhythmias, which arise below the AV junction.

Rhythm disturbances can be intermittent or established, benign or lethal and, more often than not, disturbing to the patient.

Supraventricular (SVT) arrhythmias

The impulse travels down the established pathway and characteristically produces a narrow complex. There are three exceptions, which give rise to wide QRS complexes:

* concomitant bundle branch block;
* aberration (fatigue of a bundle);
* accessory conduction (for example WPW syndrome).

Atrial ectopic beats

Atrial ectopic beats are also known as atrial premature beats, or APBs. They are characterised by premature P waves, unlike sinus P waves with an altered PR interval. The latter can be prolonged if the atrial ectopic beat encounters a refractory AV node or bundle. In atrial bigeminy every second beat is an atrial ectopic beat. In atrial trigeminy every third beat is an atrial ectopic beat.

APBs can occur in normal individuals, related to anxiety, or excessive caffeine or alcohol consumption, or they may reflect cardiac pathologies (ECGs 167–173). Treatment when indicated includes beta-blockers, verapamil, disopyramide, and sotalol.

Atrial parasystole is rare. Independent P waves are seen and the parasystolic P wave intervals have a mathematical relationship.

Supraventricular arrhythmias can be caused by:
* a re-entry mechanism;
* abnormal atrial activity.

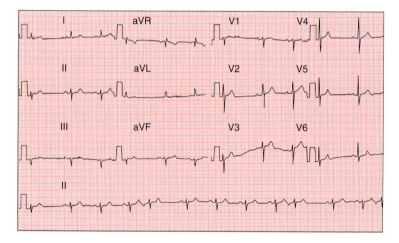

ECG 167: *This 62-year-old woman presented complaining of palpitation. The rhythm strip at the bottom of the ECG shows atrial ectopic activity in lead II. Atrial ectopic beats are characterised by inverted or altered P waves followed by a compensatory pause. This patient consumed 12 cups of strong tea per day (NB; 4/3/96).*

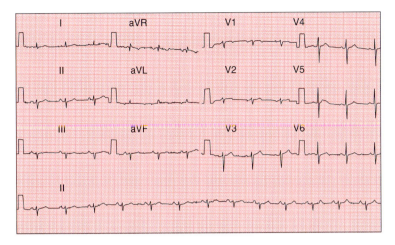

ECG 168: *After discontinuing tea, there is no further palpitation and only sinus rhythm is evident (NB; 15/4/96).*

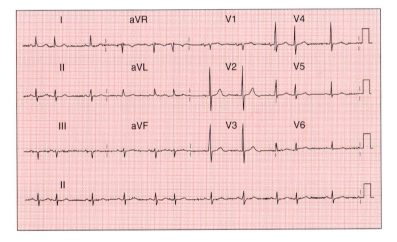

ECG 169: *An elderly man with ischaemic heart disease suffered chronic atrial extrasystoles. There was no change over the years and no attempt at medication. The atrial ectopic beats are best seen in lead II. The P wave is different to that of the sinus beats. There is a compensatory pause (RW; 29/10/99).*

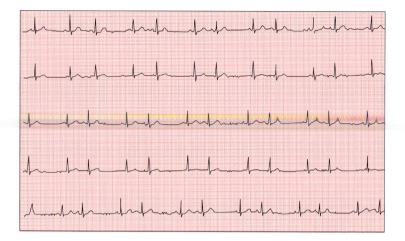

ECG 170: *24-hour Holter monitoring showing atrial ectopic beats. Every second beat is an atrial extrasystole, hence the rhythm is described as atrial bigeminy.*

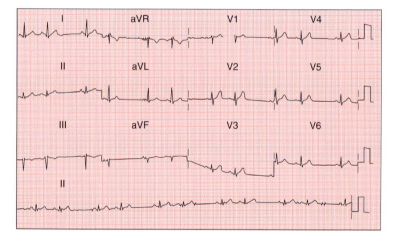

ECG 171: *A further example of atrial bigeminy (NT; 24/10/85).*

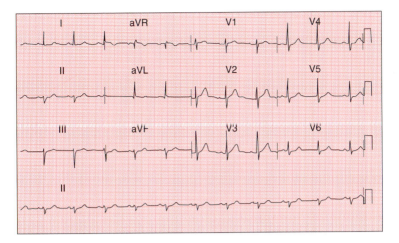

ECG 172: *Preoperative ECG from an elderly man undergoing knee replacement (RB; 1/6/99).*

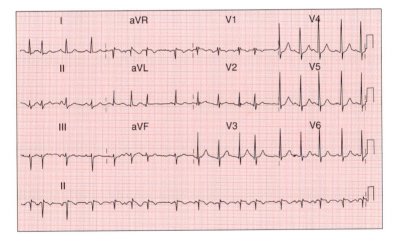

ECG 173: *Immediate postoperative ECG showing atrial ectopic activity. The patient responded to metoprolol (RB; 6/6/99).*

Re-entry mechanism

Atrioventricular nodal re-entrant (AVNR) tachycardia

This accounts for more than 50% of all SVT arrhythmias. Two functional conducting pathways are demonstrable electrophysiologically **within the AV node**: fast and slow. During sinus conduction the impulse travels down the fast pathway. Simultaneous conduction occurs down the slow pathway, but is blocked (concealed) by retrograde activation of the slow pathway, caused by the antegrade impulse travelling through the AV node. The two impulses collide and only the fast pathway is able to conduct.

AV nodal re-entrant tachycardia is defined as **common** when the re-entry circuit conducts down the slow pathway and returns via the fast pathway. P waves are not usually visible as they coincide with the QRS complex and the arrhythmia is commonly triggered by an atrial premature beat (APB). Common AVNR tachycardia is illustrated in ECGs 174–177.

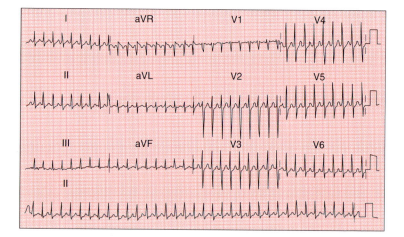

ECG 174: *This young female patient has AV nodal re-entrant tachycardia (common). The heart rate is just over 180 beats per minute, the complexes are narrow, the RR interval is regular and there are no visible P waves (AB; 12/1/93).*

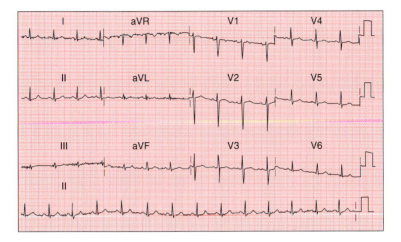

ECG 175: *The patient underwent radiofrequency ablation. She had no further symptoms. This ECG, taken 2½ years later, shows normal sinus conduction. The axis remains unchanged, confirming the supraventricular origin of the initial tachycardia (AB; 21/7/95).*

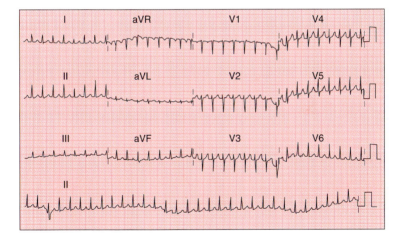

ECG 176: *This young female patient had a frequent history of palpitation. AV nodal re-entrant tachycardia is present; the heart rate is 170 beats per minute. P waves are not visible (SA; 23/6/99).*

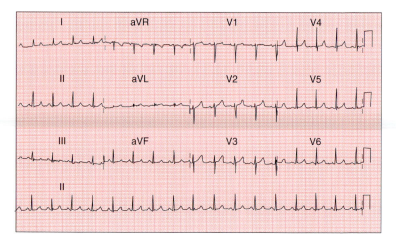

ECG 177: ECG from the same patient, taken half an hour after administration of adenosine. There is normal sinus conduction. The patient subsequently underwent ablation (AS; 23/6/99).

Uncommon AVNR tachycardia occurs in only 10% of cases. The antegrade conduction travels down the fast pathway and retrogradely up the slow pathway. Usually retrograde late P waves are seen in the inferior leads (ECGs 178 and 179). This form of SVT arrhythmia is characteristically triggered by a ventricular premature beat (VPB).

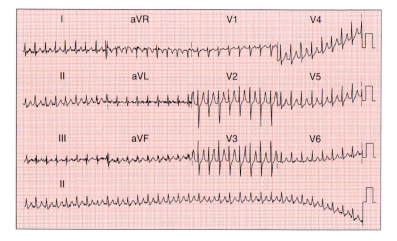

ECG 178: This 77-year-old woman has supraventricular tachycardia (AV nodal re-entry tachycardia). This is the uncommon variety, with retrograde P waves in lead V1. The heart rate is 180 beats per minute (23/10/97).

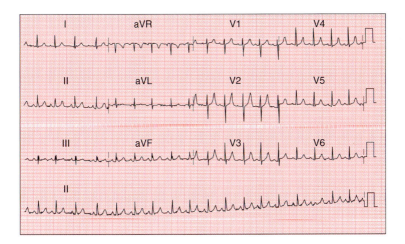

ECG 179: *ECG from the same patient 20 minutes later, after administration of intravenous adenosine; the pattern has reversed to normal sinus conduction (23/10/97).*

Atrioventricular re-entrant tachycardia

Atrioventricular re-entrant tachycardia occurs at a heart rate of 130–250 beats per minute. It is the most common form of SVT arrhythmia after AVNR tachycardia. One or more accessory pathways consisting of **extra bands of conducting tissue**, connect the atria and ventricles, for example in WPW syndrome. An APB or VPB can set off a re-entry SVT arrhythmia. The impulse travels antegradely down the normal pathway (through the AV node) and retrogradely to the atrium along the accessory pathway. No delta waves appear as conduction occurs normally. This is known as **orthodromic** atrio-ventricular re-entrant tachycardia.

In 10% of patients with WPW syndrome and AV re-entrant tachycardia the impulse travels down the accessory pathway and retrogradely through the bundle branches, the bundle of His and the AV nodal system. This is referred to as **antidromic** atrioventricular re-entrant tachycardia. It is characterised by wide QRS complexes (with exaggerated delta waves). Examples of atrioventricular re-entrant tachycardia are shown in ECGs 180–183.

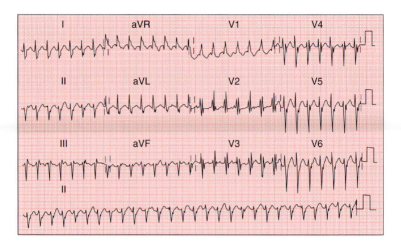

ECG 180: *ECG from a young man with regular tachycardia (150 beats per minute) with right bundle branch block. The bottom rhythm strip show retrograde P waves on the upslope of the S wave in lead II. This is probably AV re-entrant tachycardia (FC; 23/7/88).*

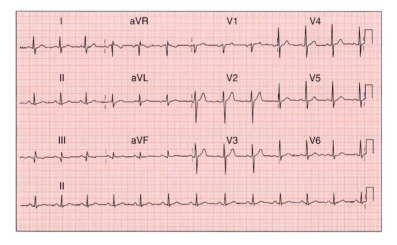

ECG 181: *ECG from the same patient 11 years later, by which time he was receiving medication. Note the change of axis and bundle branch block (aberration) during tachycardia in ECG 180 (FC; 20/1/99).*

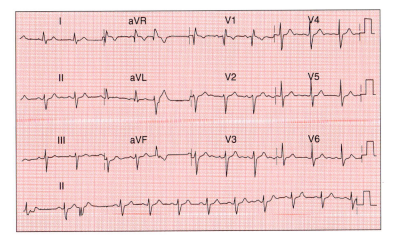

ECG 182: *Preoperative ECG showing sinus rhythm, right bundle branch block and left axis deviation. (HB; 4/3/96).*

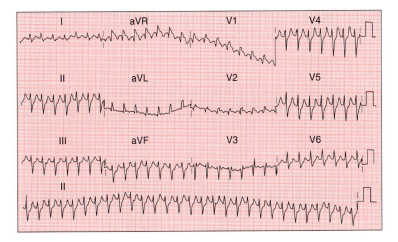

ECG 183: *Perioperative ECG showing rapid supraventricular arrhythmia. The complexes are wide because of the underlying right bundle branch block; the heart rate is 150 beats per minute. The patient made a spontaneous recovery (HB; 8/3/96).*

Abnormal atrial activity

Junctional tachycardia

In junctional tachycardia there is enhanced automaticity or triggered activity within the AV junction (not re-entry), a rare cause of SVT in adults. The condition occurs in the presence of trauma to the AV junction (for example surgery, digoxin toxicity, acute myocardial infarction). Characteristically, the SVT produces a narrow complex showing AV dissociation or 1:1 ventricular atrial activation (ECGs 184–188).

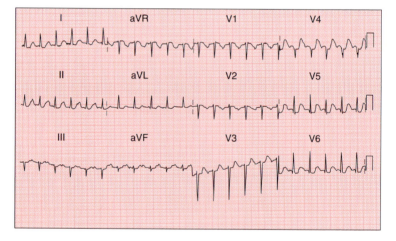

ECG 184: *Probable junctional tachycardia. Retrograde P waves are best seen in lead III and aVF. Rate 128 beats/minute (SV; 20/6/99).*

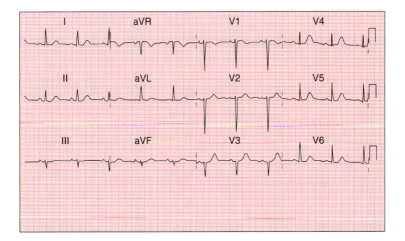

ECG 185: *ECG from the same patient taken the next day, after medication (SV; 21/6/99).*

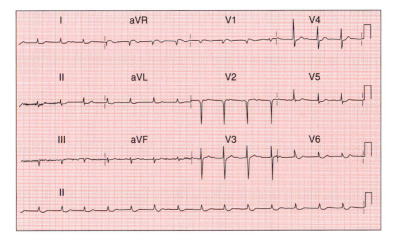

ECG 186: *Junctional rhythm. The complexes are narrow and the rhythm is regular. There are no visible P waves. The patient is elderly, postoperative and died soon after this trace was taken (RG; 2/11/99).*

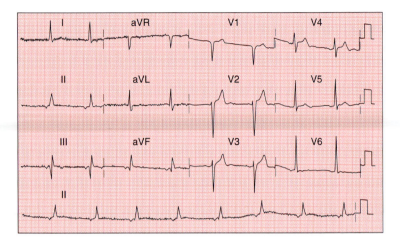

ECG 187: *AV junctional rhythm (coronary sinus rhythm). There are inverted P waves leads II, III and aVF. This patient had previously undergone bypass surgery (AB; 21/7/95).*

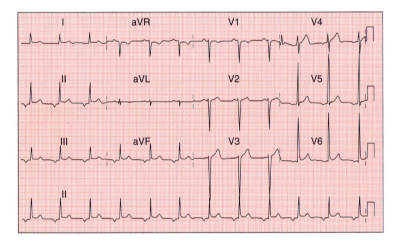

ECG 188: *A further example of atrioventricular junctional rhythm. The diagnosis is mitral valve prolapse (PJ; 6/10/97).*

Atrial tachycardia (rate 120–250 bpm)

Unifocal

The P wave is of single morphological pattern. The atrial rate is usually below 250 beats per minute. The arrhythmia originates in atrial musculature; the mechanism can involve a re-entry circuit, or enhanced automaticity, or triggered activity such as in digoxin toxicity (ECG

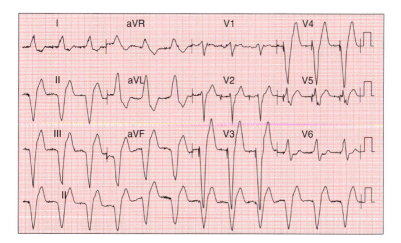

ECG 189: *Dual chamber pacing. Atrial and ventricular pacing signals are seen clearly in lead V1 and V2 (SB; 20/4/98).*

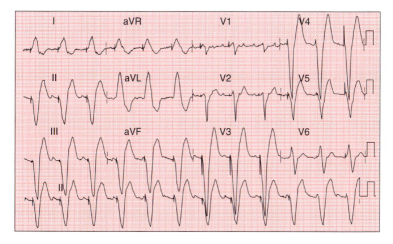

ECG 190: *The same patient developed an atrial tachycardia. P waves are seen clearly in lead V1. P rate is 180 beats per minute (atrial tachycardia P rate is usually between 120 and 250 beats per minute) (SB; 11/8/99).*

190). This is a rare cause of SVT arrhythmia. It can occur in the presence of heart disease, but does not necessarily do so.

Multifocal

P waves of varying morphology are recognisable. This arrhythmia is rare; it is seen in acutely ill patients, often with underlying pulmonary disease.

Atrial flutter

Typical (Type I)

Typical atrial flutter is caused by a re-entrant counterclockwise macro-circuit in the right atrium. Negative saw-toothed F waves are seen in inferior leads. The atrial rate averages 300 beats per minute. If the F waves are positive in the inferior leads, the macrocircuit conducts clockwise.

Atypical (Type II)

The atrial rate is faster than in typical atrial flutter, at up to 400 beats per minute, with positive deflections in the inferior leads. Atypical flutter can conduct with 2:1 or 4:1 heart block or variable block, depending on the refractory properties of the conducting system. If the block is variable the pulse will be irregular, hence the necessity of ECG documentation. Causes of atrial flutter include hyperthyroidism, ischaemic heart disease, hypertension, rheumatic heart disease, cardiomyopathies, pericarditis, congenital heart conditions, pulmonary disease, sick sinus syndrome and drug abuse, particularly alcohol.

Examples of ECG appearance in patients with atrial flutter are shown in ECGs 191–215.

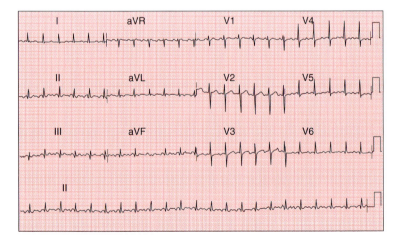

ECG 191: *Perioperative ECG (after bypass surgery) showing rapid tachycardia at 140 beats per minute. Note the narrow complexes. Flutter waves are seen in rhythm strip II, occurring at 300 beats per minute. The diagnosis is atrial flutter (JB; 20/6/99).*

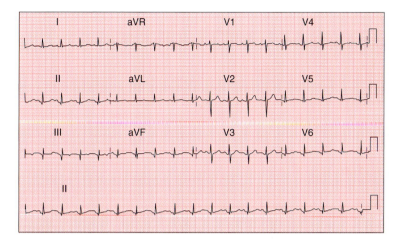

ECG 192: *ECG from the same patient after medication, 2 hours later (JB; 20/6/99).*

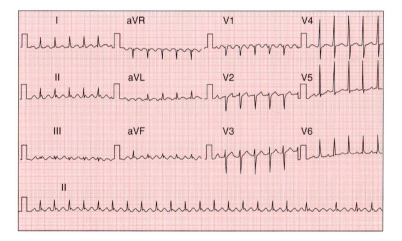

ECG 193: *Classical atrial flutter. The seesaw appearance is present in lead II. Flutter waves are occurring at ± 300 beats per minute with a ventricular rate of 142 beats per minute, in other words a 2:1 response. At the end of the rhythm strip (bottom line) there is more profound block. The ventricular rate slows down, but the flutter waves are unaltered (ET; 9/1/95).*

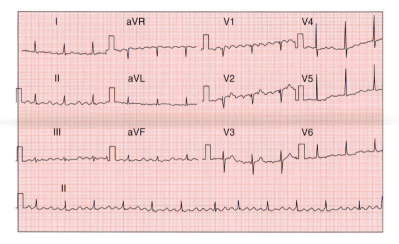

ECG 194: *The same patient 2 months later, on digoxin, has converted to atrial fibrillation. The QRS complexes are now occurring irregularly (ET; 6/3/95).*

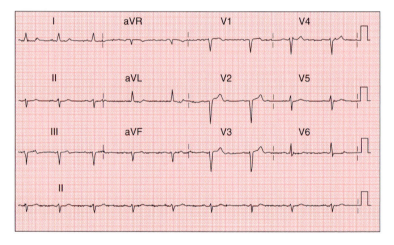

ECG 195: *An elderly patient who had undergone bypass surgery shows sinus rhythm, anteroseptal Q waves and left axis deviation (HI; 10/11/98).*

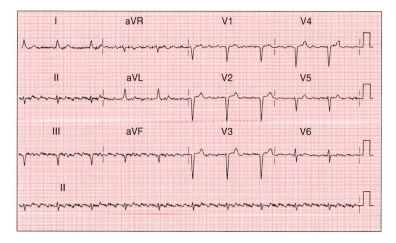

ECG 196: *The same patient presented with abnormal rhythm several months later. There is no change in the QRS complexes or axis. The ventricular rate is 60 beats per minute. There are P waves (best seen in lead V1), occurring at a rate of 190 beats per minute. Rhythm strip II at the bottom of the ECG would suggest an atrial flutter, but the P rate is too slow. The diagnosis is more likely an atrial tachycardia (HI; 5/1/99).*

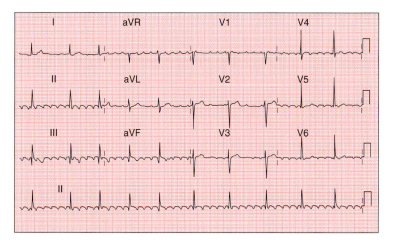

ECG 197: *Atrial flutter. The P rate is 300 beats per minute, and the ventricular rate is 56 beats per minute. This is atrial flutter with 4:1 AV block (AC; 7/4/97).*

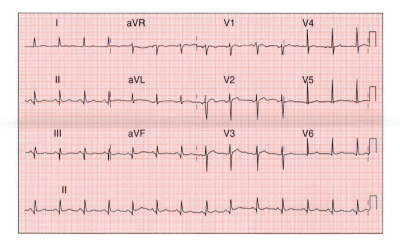

ECG 198: *The same patient was in sinus rhythm several months later. Inferior Q waves are more clearly visible. They can also be appreciated during the flutter episode (AC; 23/6/97).*

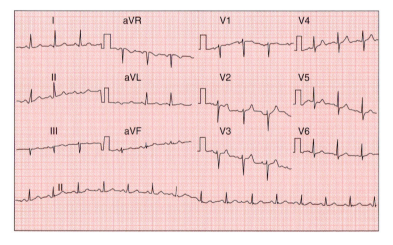

ECG 199: *Normal sinus conduction (R McL; 22/1/96).*

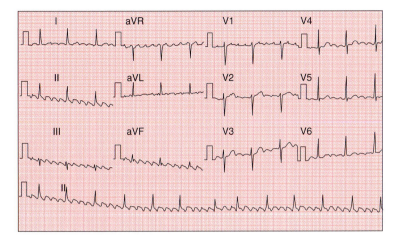

ECG 200: *Nine months later there is atrial flutter, with a ventricular rate of 70 beats per minute. The flutter rate is 300 beats per minute. Rhythm strip lead II at the bottom of the ECG shows variable AV block, with a characteristic seesaw appearance (R McL; 21/10/96).*

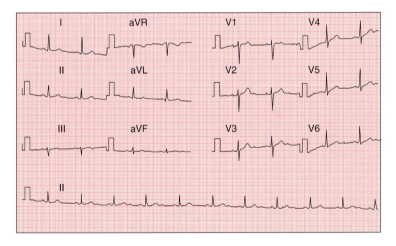

ECG 201: *Normal sinus conduction is evident 2 months later, after successful cardioversion (R McL; 9/12/96).*

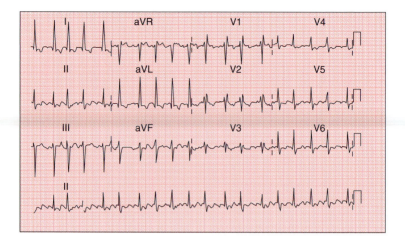

ECG 202: ECG from a 40-year-old patient after aortic valve replacement. There is atrial flutter, P wave activity at 300 beats per minute, and variable AV block (PL; 15/6/99).

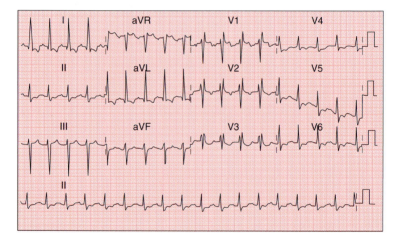

ECG 203: The same patient immediately after cardioversion. Sinus rhythm is reestablished. There are upright P waves in lead I, and negative P waves in lead V1 (PL; 15/6/99).

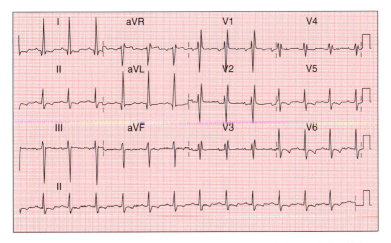

ECG 204: *Two months later sinus rhythm is maintained. Note right bundle branch block and left ventricle voltages (PL; 8/9/99).*

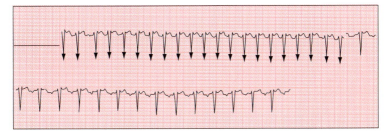

ECG 205: *The same patient showing a flutter rhythm at cardioversion. The initial rate is 158 beats per minute. The thick arrows indicate a synchronised signal from the cardioversion apparatus. Immediately after cardioversion, the rate is just over 90 beats per minute and inverted P waves are clearly visible (PL; 15/6/99).*

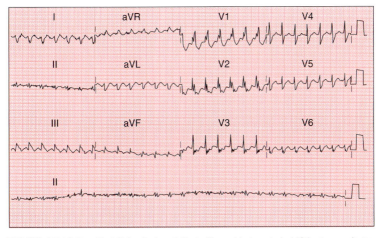

ECG 206: *Atrial flutter with right bundle branch block. The ventricular rate is 140 beats per minute; flutter waves are occurring at 300 beats per minute. The seesaw appearance is evident in lead III (HB; 2/5/96).*

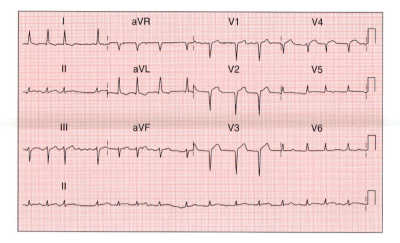

ECG 207: Middle-aged patient after bypass surgery showing atrial fibrillation (AL; 16/6/98).

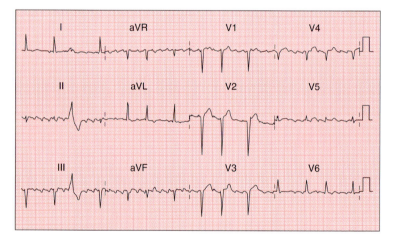

ECG 208: On medication, atrial flutter waves develop (at 300 beats per minute); these are best seen in leads II and aVR (AL; 20/6/98).

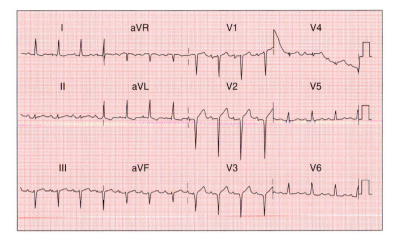

ECG 209: *The patient was restored to sinus rhythm after successful cardioversion. P waves in leads II, III and aVF are notched, indicating high left atrial pressure (AL; 20/6/98).*

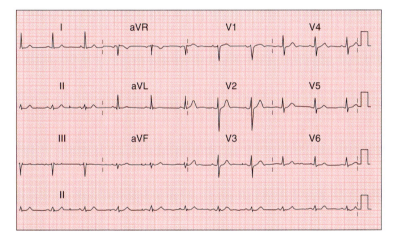

ECG 210: *ECG from a middle-aged patient, years after bypass surgery (ED; 28/7/98).*

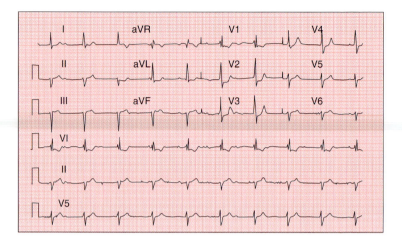

ECG 211: *During bladder surgery, the patient suffer a perioperative inferior infarction. Ventricular rate is 57 beats per minute. Dissociated P waves are seen best in leads I and II; there is nodal rhythm with AV dissociation (ED; 3/8/98).*

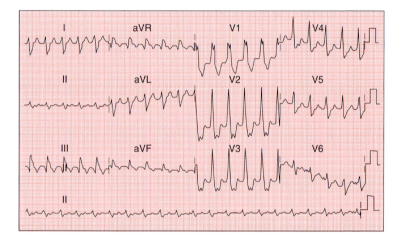

ECG 212: *The same patient, 2 months later. The ECG shows tachycardia and a ventricular rate of 120 beats per minute causing right bundle branch block (aberration). Leads III and aVF suggest atrial flutter; atrial activity is 180 beats per minute (ED; 2/10/98).*

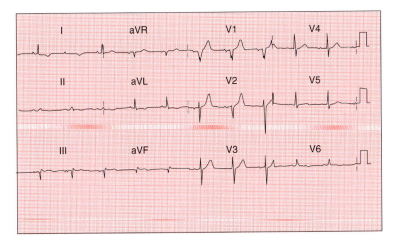

ECG 213: *Two days later the patient is back to sinus conduction (with medication) with normal QRS complexes. Residual Q waves are visible in leads III and AVF (ED; 4/10/98).*

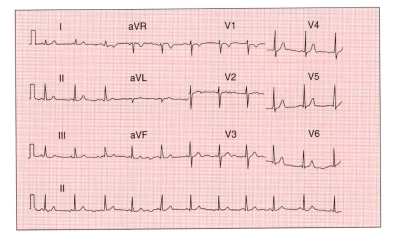

ECG 214: *Normal electrocardiogram in a young Japanese patient (MS; 13/2/93).*

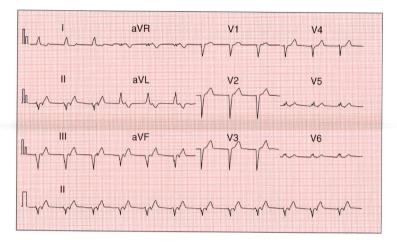

ECG 215: *ECG from the same patient showing nodal (junctional) rhythm, a ventricular rate of 72 beats per minute and regular, widened QRS complexes (LBBB). Retrograde P waves are seen best in the inferior leads (MS).*

Atrial fibrillation

Atrial fibrillation is the commonest of all arrhythmias. It has the same aetiology as atrial flutter, increasing in frequency with ageing. Here the atria do not contract: they 'fibrillate' at a rate of 300 to 600 beats per minute. The AV node cannot cope with this number of impulses and only some will get through to the ventricles. Atrial fibrillation is caused by multiple microwavelet re-entry circuits. Therefore the ventricular response is totally irregular. The ventricular rate is usually fast, but occasionally it is extremely slow and pacing may be required (for example in sick sinus syndrome). Rarely, atrial fibrillation can coexist with complete heart block. The ventricular rate then becomes regular and slow, the complexes are wide (originating in the ventricles), but usually the F waves are still visible. Atrial flutter or AV nodal re-entrant tachycardia can degenerate to atrial fibrillation. Lone atrial fibrillation refers to arrhythmia for which no cause can be detected. ECGs 216–243 illustrate the different appearances of atrial fibrillation.

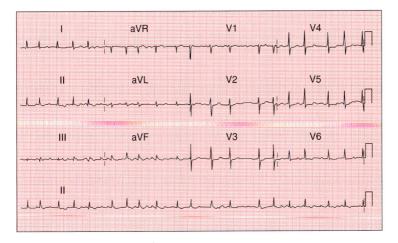

ECG 216: *ECG from a middle-aged man with ischaemic heart disease. There is paroxysmal atrial fibrillation and the ventricular rate is irregular with classical 'fibrillatory waves' in lead V1 (AS; 4/6/98).*

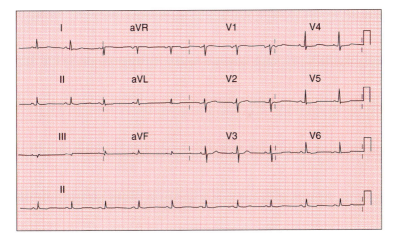

ECG 217: *The same patient after electrical cardioversion. There is sinus rhythm with similar complexes and axis (AS; 15/6/98).*

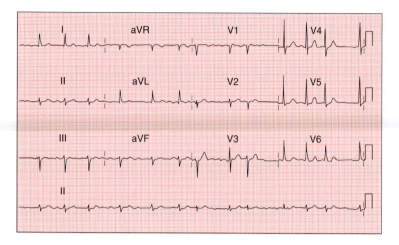

ECG 218: Atrial fibrillation of recent onset in a middle-aged man who had consumed an excessive amount of alcohol (SG; 25/3/98).

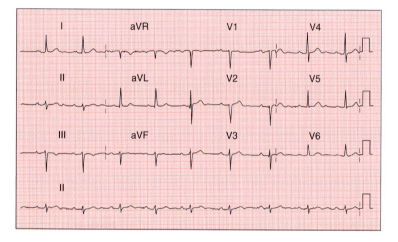

ECG 219: After failed medical conversion with amiodarone and digoxin the patient is successfully restored to sinus rhythm with electrical cardioversion (SG; 19/5/98).

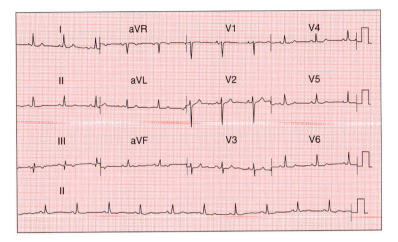

ECG 220: *ECG from an elderly woman with ischaemic heart disease (KF; 11/3/93).*

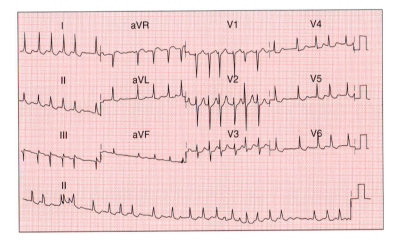

ECG 221: *The patient was admitted in rapid atrial fibrillation, with a ventricular rate of 150–170 beats per minute. The tachycardia gives rise to angina, and digoxin induced ST changes are also visible. The third 'complex' in the rhythm strip is an artefact (KF; 9/1/93).*

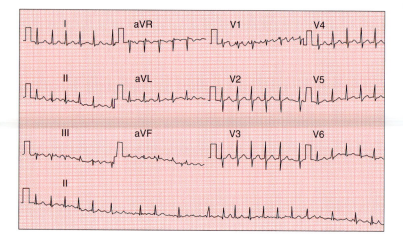

ECG 222: *Rapid atrial fibrillation in a middle-aged man. The patient had no symptoms and no cause for atrial fibrillation was found (Mr H; 21/2/97).*

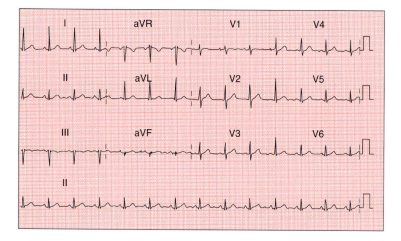

ECG 223: *The same patient 18 months later, in sinus rhythm (Mr H; 19/8/98).*

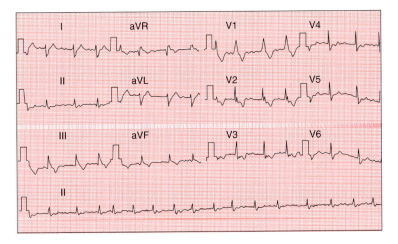

ECG 224: *This elderly man had established atrial fibrillation. There is right bundle branch block, with right axis deviation constituting a bifascicular block (AS; 6/12/96).*

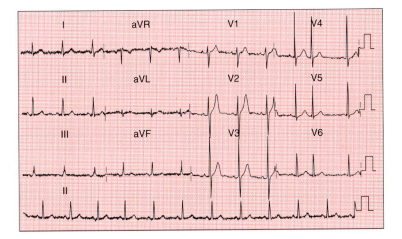

ECG 225: *ECG from a middle-aged man with previous rheumatic mitral disease and mitral valvotomy. Sinus rhythm is evident (SC; 23/6/93).*

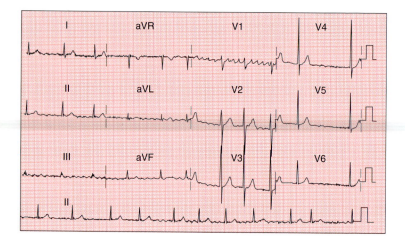

ECG 226: Coarse atrial fibrillation is evident 2 years later (SC; 8/4/95).

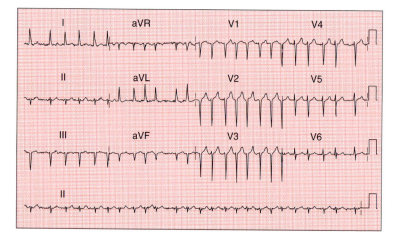

ECG 227: Rapid atrial fibrillation. There are narrow complexes, an irregular ventricular response and a ventricular rate of 156 beats per minute. There are no P waves (FJ; 12/6/99).

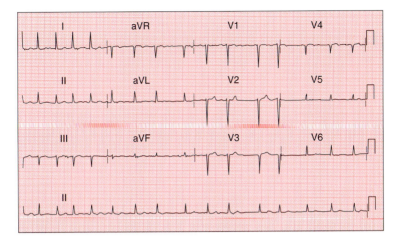

ECG 228: *This elderly woman with stable angina presented with atrial fibrillation that was controlled medically (Mr H; 4/6/98).*

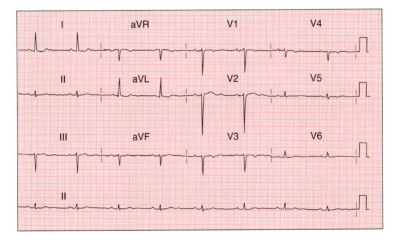

ECG 229: *Three weeks later there is medical cardioversion to sinus rhythm. Note similarity of complexes and electric axis (MH; 30/6/98).*

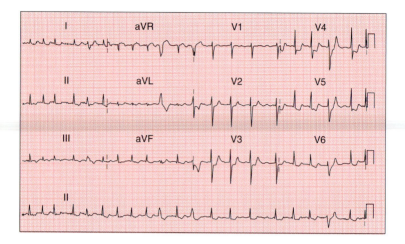

ECG 230: Episodic atrial fibrillation in an elderly patient with ischaemic heart disease and a dual chamber pacemaker. Atrial fibrillation causes marked precordial ischaemic changes. Pacing is inhibited by the ventricular rate (SB; 15/6/98).

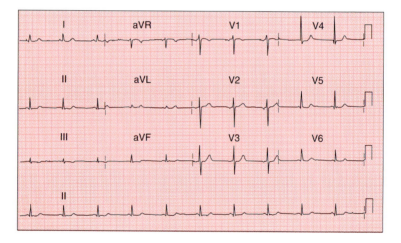

ECG 231: Two weeks later there is medical cardioversion. A pacing signal is seen in lead V1. There are no significant ischaemic changes (SB; 1/7/98).

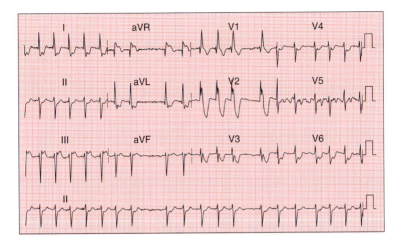

ECG 232: *ECG from an elderly lady 10 years after bypass surgery. There is sudden onset of atrial fibrillation, with marked ischaemic changes in leads I, aVL and V6, and right bundle branch block. The trace shows left axis deviation (bifascicular block) (SB; 25/9/99).*

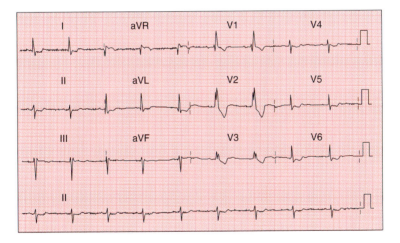

ECG 233: *Reversal with oral amiodarone 24 hours later. The patient is restored to sinus rhythm; there is right bundle branch block with minimal anterolateral ST ischaemic changes (SB; 26/9/99).*

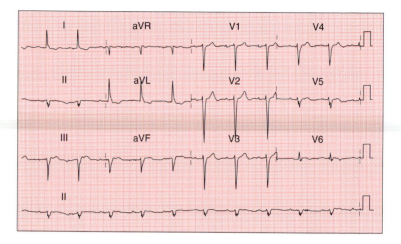

ECG 234: *ECG from a middle-aged woman with silent inferior infarction. There is normal sinus conduction with widened QRS complexes (intraventricular conduction defect) (Mrs J; 11/11/97).*

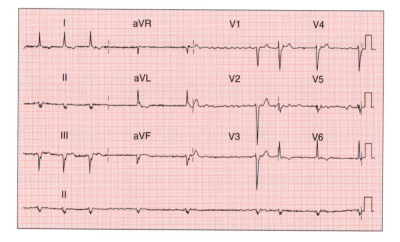

ECG 235: *Six months later there is onset of very slow atrial fibrillation. The remaining ECG pattern is unchanged. The patient was successfully restored to sinus rhythm with electrical cardioversion (Mrs J; 26/5/98).*

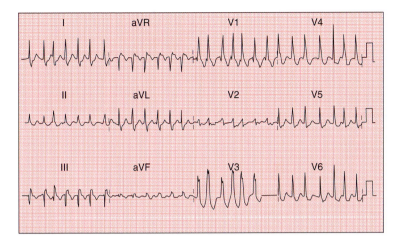

ECG 236: *Broad spectrum tachycardia. This could be confused with ventricular tachycardia (Mr K; 14/7/98).*

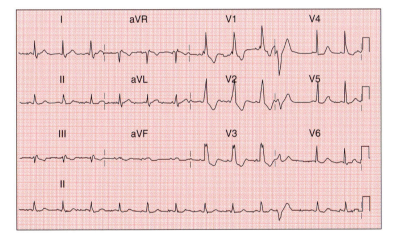

ECG 237: *ECG from the same patient showing sinus rhythm with right bundle branch block. The diagnosis is atrial fibrillation (Mr K).*

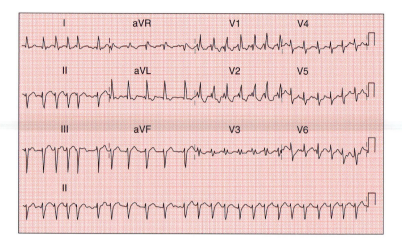

ECG 238: *This 82-year-old patient was admitted in rapid atrial fibrillation with right bundle branch block and left axis deviation. The ventricular rate is clearly irregular. Medication was instituted with amiodarone. The patient was already on atenolol, digoxin and verapamil (SF; 14/10/98).*

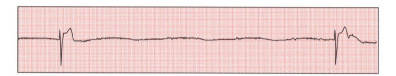

ECG 239: *The effect of overmedication. There is ventricular asystole and P waves are just discernible (10/10/98).*

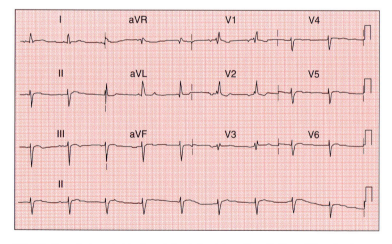

ECG 240: *The patient reverted to sinus rhythm 4 days later, without ill effects. This series shows that accumulative antiarrhythmics can have profound negative chronotropic effects (SF; 7/10/98).*

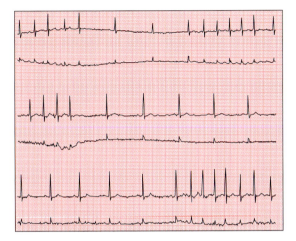

ECG 241: *24-hour ambulatory Holter monitoring showing classical so-called sick sinus syndrome (tachycardia/bradycardic).*

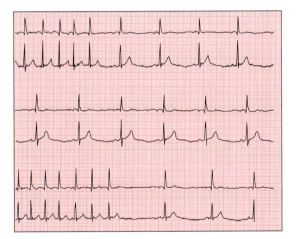

ECG 242: *These continuous strips show the patient going from fairly rapid atrial fibrillation into sudden sinus bradycardia.*

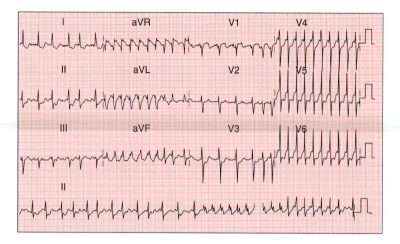

ECG 243: *Rapid atrial fibrillation with marked lateral ischaemic changes. The rhythm strip at the bottom (lead II) shows a short run of bundle branch block. This is a rare dependent aberration (Mrs L; 6/5/93).*

Left untreated, these supraventricular arrhythmias can bring on congestive cardiac failure with dilatation of the heart, which is more likely in patients with underlying cardiac pathologies. Atrial fibrillation poses a significant risk: emboli can occur and can pass to the lungs from the right atrium, or to the systemic circulation from the left atrium or rarely, across a patent foramen (paradoxical emboli). The prevalence of atrial fibrillation is 0.5% in people aged 50-59 years, rising to 8.8% in people aged 80-89 years. There is a six-fold increase in thromboembolic phenomena (5% per annum). It is known that 36% of strokes in the elderly are the result of atrial fibrillation. Cardiac output is reduced from between 25% to 50%, giving rise to symptoms of fatigue and breathlessness.

Proper anticoagulation with warfarin reduces the risk of stroke by up to 70%. The target is an international ratio (INR; a measure of prothrombin time) of 2.0-2.5 and so warfarin is the drug of choice, even in the elderly, although aspirin can be used in low risk patients (those with normal left atrial dimension, no congestive cardiac failure or mitral disease).

The aim of treatment is to restore sinus rhythm if possible. This can be done medically or by electrical cardioversion. Ideally the patient should be given warfarin for at least 3 weeks and started on oral amiodarone with a loading dose (200 mg tid) for several days, continuing with 200 mg daily for up to 4 weeks. The success rate is variable. The best results are obtained with recently developed atrial fibrillation in the presence of normal left ventricular function and normal left atrial dimension (4 cm) on echocardiography. IV flecainide is also useful, but is to be avoided after acute myocardial infarction.

Electric cardioversion is the next step. The patient's INR should be between 2.0 and 2.5. The usual starting output is 200 Joules, moving up to 360 Joules. Several shocks may have to be administered under acting general anaesthesia. Warfarin should be continued for at least 3 weeks. There is some evidence that atrial 'stunning' persists so that late emboli can occur. In dire emergencies, when anticoagulation with warfarin is not possible, an intravenous bolus of 5000 units of heparin should be administered half an hour before electric cardioversion.

Pharmacological management of SVT arrhythmias

The indications and dosages of antiarrhythmic agents are summarised in Tables 1 and 2 on pages 228–30.

Acute

Supraventricular re-entry tachycardia
Suitable pharmacological agents include intravenous adenosine, verapamil, disopyramide, flecainide, beta-blockers (esmolol), or amiodarone through a central vein. Digoxin can be administered intra-venously (slowly) or intramuscularly. A new drug, dofetilide, has a promising profile.

Atrial flutter, fibrillation, atrial tachycardia
Treatment is the same as that for supraventricular re-entry tachycardia, with the exception of adenosine, which is not suitable.

WPW syndrome with SVT
Suitable pharmacological agents include IV flecainide, disopyramide, beta-blockers (sotalol) and amiodarone. It is important to note that verapamil and digoxin are contraindicated; they slow down AV conduction and can therefore accelerate the rhythm.

Chronic
Suitable oral preparations include digoxin, verapamil, sotalol, diso-pyramide, amiodarone, flecainide and propafenone.

Special precautions

Note that verapamil and beta-blockers slow heart rate and verapamil increases digoxin toxicity. Amiodarone can cause severe bradycardia alone or in combination with other medication (ECG 239). Warfarin will react with a number of preparations, and INR monitoring is essential.

Prevention

After successful medical or electrical cardioversion the following drugs can prevent recurrences: flecainide, sotalol, propafenone, amiodarone, and quinidine.

Quinidine was previously used regularly. It is not favoured now as it can generate a form of VT (torsade de pointes) giving rise to so-called quinidine syncope. However, it is still used in the USA, and is worth trying if all else fails. New drugs that are presently being evaluated include azimilide and dofetilide.

Mechanical management of SVT arrhythmias

DC conversion

DC conversion is covered in Chapter 8.

Implantable atrial defibrillators

Implantable atrial defibrillators will sense the onset of SVT arrhythmia and deliver a DC shock to the atrium. These devices are presently being evaluated.

Ablation

Electrophysiological study is required to map the abnormal circuits. Once established, radiofrequency energy is applied to one of the abnormal pathways, 'burning it off', and disabling the re-entry circuit. This technique is particularly useful in re-entry supraventricular tachy-cardias offering a very high percentage of cure at a very low risk.

Surgery

The 'Maze' operation involves creating 'corridors' within the atria to interfere with the propagation of the abnormal impulses. This proce-dure is more favoured in the United States.

AV nodal ablation

AV nodal ablation is useful in intractable symptomatic atrial fibrilla-tion. It requires permanent pacemaker implantation, so that patients are entirely dependent on pacing.

Pulmonary vein ablation

In some patients atrial arrhythmias originate in the pulmonary vein, where ablation can be beneficial.

Ventricular arrhythmias

Ventricular extrasystoles

Ventricular extrasystoles are also known as ventricular premature beats (VPBs). These are **broad complexes** (QRS over 120 ms) that are premature by definition (hence the compensatory pause), therefore the coupling interval (interval between ectopic and previous beat) is short. VPBs can occur in isolation arising from the right ventricle (giving rise to a left bundle branch block pattern) or the left ventricle (producing a right bundle branch block pattern). They can be benign or associated with myocardial damage (for example ischaemia, infarction, cardiomyopathies and myocarditis). They can be caused by drugs such as digoxin, antiarrhythmics, cocaine, excessive caffeine, alcohol, catecholamines (anxiety) and bronchodilators. VPBs are described as **unifocal** when they arise from a single source, all being similar in configuration, or **multifocal**, when they originate from different foci and have a varying appearance.

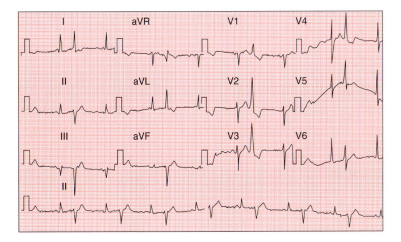

ECG 244: *Ventricular extrasystoles (or premature beats). These are clearly different to sinus beats as they originate in the ventricles as opposed to atrial extrasystoles (premature atrial beats) which would use the same conducting pathway as the sinus conducted beats. In leads V1 and V6 these extrasystoles have a right bundle branch block configuration and originate from the left ventricle. The rhythm strip at the bottom of the page shows that every second beat is a ventricular extrasystole and this would therefore be called ventricular bigeminy (HH; 27/3/95).*

Ventricular bigeminy

In ventricular bigeminy every sinus beat is followed by a ventricular extrasystole (ECG 244).

Ventricular trigeminy

In ventricular trigeminy every second sinus beat is followed by a ventricular extrasystole.

Ventricular couplets

Ventricular couplets are defined as two consecutive VPBs (ECG 245).

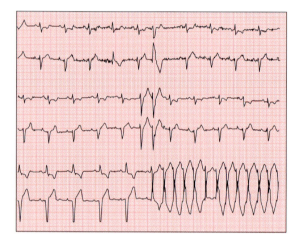

ECG 245: *24-Hour ambulatory Holter monitor traces from a patient who had undergone bypass surgery. The two simultaneous channels in the upper strip show one ventricular extrasystole in the middle followed by a compensatory pause. The middle strip shows two consecutive ventricular extrasystoles. This is a ventricular couplet. The bottom strip shows a run of normal sinus rhythm with a ventricular extrasystole falling just at the end of the T wave of the sinus beat, setting off a run of ventricular tachycardia (MS).*

Ventricular salvo

Ventricular salvo constitutes more than two consecutive VPBs.

Ventricular parasystole

Ventricular parasystole is uncommon. VPBs occur regularly and are not related to the dominant rhythm. This syndrome is characterised by variable coupling intervals, mathematically related RR intervals and the presence of fusion beats. No treatment is indicated.

Management of ventricular premature beats

If there is no underlying cardiac pathology VPBs are best ignored. The patient should be advised to reduce consumption of caffeine, bronchodilators, alcohol and tobacco. In the presence of unpleasant symptoms a course of mexilitene, disopyramide, flecainide or propafenone is recommended. All can prove beneficial. If innocent, VPBs usually disappear during a stress test. In the presence of underlying cardiac pathology (for example metabolic disorders, drug overdose, or acidosis) treat accordingly. If VPBs are related to ischaemic heart disease (indicated by worsening during a stress test), they may respond to anginal medication. Particular care is required after myocardial infarction as ventricular extrasystoles may herald ventricular tachycardia; this responds to intravenous lignocaine. If VPBs are related to dilated cardiomyopathy or congestive cardiac failure, amiodarone becomes the drug of choice (it has no negative inotropic effect).

Ventricular tachycardia (VT)

These are broad complex tachycardias arising from the right or left ventricles with QRS complex duration usually over 120 milliseconds. Most are caused by re-entry mechanisms, some from enhanced automaticity. They can be sustained (lasting over 30 seconds) or non-sustained. They are described as monomorphic when each complex has the same configuration or polymorphic when the QRS pattern twists across the baseline (torsade de pointes). VT can degenerate into VF, particularly in the context of acute myocardial infarction, with lethal consequences. However, there are also benign ventricular tachycardias.

In ventricular tachycardia, atrial activity remains unaffected, hence it is imperative to obtain 12 lead ECGs during an attack. The P waves will be generally of a slower rate compared to the ventricular arrhythmia. They appear independently (AV dissociation), at regular intervals, and are distinctly recognisable, deforming QRS or T waves when they coincide. Retrograde P waves are seen when the ventricle activates the atria. As this can occur in up to 45% of cases of VT, AV dissociation is clearly not invariable. Fusion beats (simultaneous activation when atrial and ventricular impulses coincide) or captured beats (when the atrial stimulus captures the AV node and stimulates the ventricles during a VT) also point to a diagnosis of ventricular tachycardia. Examples of ventricular tachycardia are shown in ECGs 246–254.

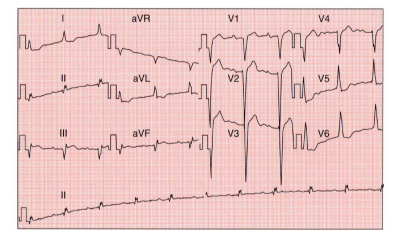

ECG 246: 24-Hour Holter monitor trace. At the bottom of the continuous strip, a ventricular extrasystole occurs at the end of a sinus T wave, setting off a run of ventricular tachycardia. The patient is in AF.

ECG 247: ECG trace showing sinus rhythm, left bundle branch block, a prolonged PR interval and inferior Q waves (WL; 1980s).

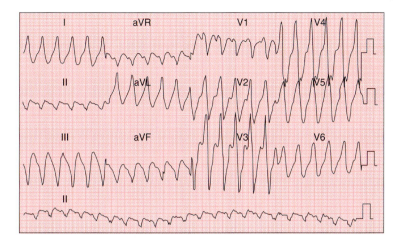

ECG 248: *The same patient developed ventricular tachycardia. The patient had bypass surgery and developed ischaemic cardiomyopathy and eventually died as a result of VT/VF. Here the VT occurred after treatment with flecainide (pro-arrhythmic effect) (WL; April 1990).*

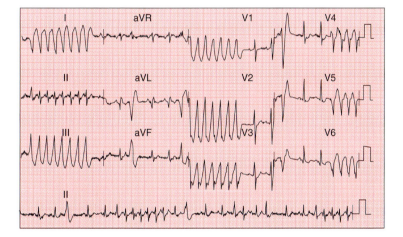

ECG 249: *This patient presented with syncopal attacks caused by runs of self-remitting (non-sustained) ventricular tachycardia. He had a myocardial infarction many years previously. After electrophysiological study he was treated medically with amiodarone and metoprolol (JG; 30/12/92).*

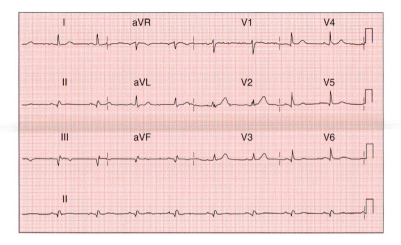

ECG 250: *The same patient 6 years later is in sinus rhythm with old inferior Q wave infarction. He had no further symptoms on this regimen. Note the prolonged QT interval caused by medication (JG; 7/10/98).*

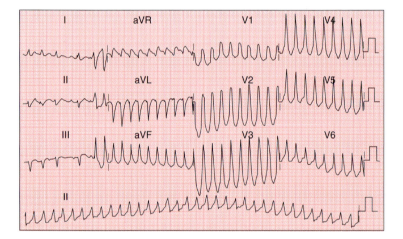

ECG 251: *ECG from an 89-year-old woman with ischaemic heart disease and chronic congestive cardiac failure showing ventricular tachycardia treated medically. Note that the patient is in sinus rhythm at the beginning of the trace. P waves are seen clearly in lead II. Ventricular tachycardia develops during the recording. Note the different rhythm strip from lead II at the bottom of the page. The run of VT shows so-called concordance. All the precordial leads show a similar axis. This is pathognomonic of ventricular tachycardia (EL; 10/10/89).*

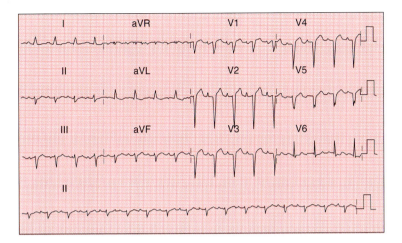

ECG 252: *Four days later a routine ECG shows sinus conduction with widespread anterolateral Q waves (EL; 14/10/89).*

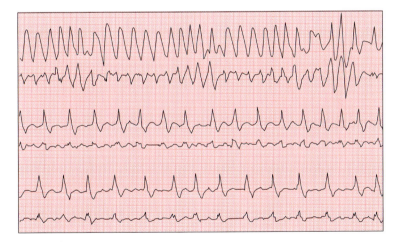

ECG 253: *Non-sustained ventricular tachycardia recorded on a 24-hour tape. The patient spontaneously returns to sinus conduction.*

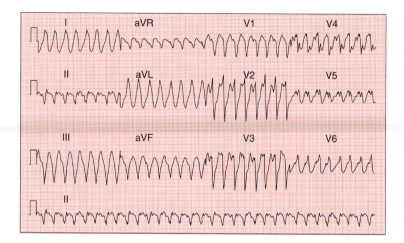

ECG 254: ECG taken during ventricular tachycardia. There are wide QRS complexes. Retrograde P waves are seen in lead V1 independent of ventricular activity (CG; 12/4/99).

Other useful pointers

* Left rabbit ear: the R wave in V1 is taller than the R' wave.
* Concordance: can be positive or negative when all complexes in the precordial leads point either up or down.
* As a general rule, 90% of broad complex tachycardias (QRS complexes over 120 ms), will be ventricular tachycardias.
* Wide QRS complexes can also occur with:
  1) bundle branch block or aberration
  2) an accessory pathway (e.g. WPW syndrome)
  3) slow conduction through the bundle of His and Purkinje system (toxic, metabolic myocardial damage).

Causes of ventricular tachycardia

Ventricular tachycardia is usually caused by organic heart disease, most commonly after acute myocardial infarction. In addition, it can occur in chronic ischaemic heart disease, left ventricular aneurysm, cardiomyopathies (dilated and hypertrophic), myocarditis related to drugs or as a result of antiarrhythmic medication (proarrhythmia). It can be related to hypokalaemia, low serum magnesium, hypoxia, or catecholamines (bronchodilators). Frequent ventricular premature beats often herald the development of ventricular tachycardia, particularly in acute ischaemic situations.

Specific ventricular tachycardias

Slow VT or accelerated idioventricular rhythm

Slow VT is seen after acute myocardial infarction. The ventricular rate is usually below 120 beats per minute, and is monomorphic. AV dissociation is evident. The condition is benign and self-remitting; no treatment is indicated.

Right ventricular outflow tract tachycardia

The condition is not generally dangerous, is exercised induced and usually not sustained. It is a re-entrant tachycardia that originates in the right ventricular outflow tract without obvious underlying pathology. Right ventricular outflow tract tachycardia is characterised by left bundle branch block and right axis deviation. Treatment is with beta-blockers or ablation.

Fascicular ventricular tachycardia

Fascicular ventricular tachycardia is uncommon, usually arising from the posterior fascicle of the left bundle, but occasionally from the anterior fascicle. There is no evidence of underlying heart disease. It affects young people, is exercise induced and re-entrant. Posterior fascicle ventricular tachycardia is characterised by right bundle branch block with left axis deviation and that which arises from the anterior fascicle produces a right bundle branch block with right axis deviation. Treatment is with verapamil or ablation.

Arrhythmogenic right ventricular dysplasia

The condition occurs in the presence of a dilated right ventricle caused by lack of muscle fibres (for example Uhl's syndrome). There is a left bundle branch pattern. It effects young people and is exercise related.

Torsade de pointes

Torsade de pointes produces an ECG that is polymorphic, undulating, and associated with a prolonged QT interval (ECG 255).

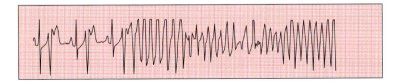

ECG 255: *Torsade de pointes. Note the 'undulating' effect.*

Prolonged QT interval

Acquired

An acquired prolonged QT interval is associated with certain drugs, for example quinidine, disopyramide, amiodarone and sotalol. It can be associated with bradycardia (for example in sick sinus syndrome or AV block). In addition, it can be seen with hypokalaemia, hypomagnesaemia and rarely with erythromycin, or tricyclic antidepressants. Treatment is by withdrawal of the culprit drug, and avoiding bradycardia. Magnesium can be given as 2 g (20 ml or 10% solution) intravenously over 2 minutes or by a continuous infusion of 3–10 mg/min. DC defibrillation is indicated if ventricular fibrillation develops.

Congenital

Congenital prolonged QT intervals occur in Romano–Ward syndrome and Jervell–Lange–Nielson syndrome. Treatment is with beta-blockers, magnesium, and pacing.

Symptoms of ventricular tachycardia

These are cerebral consisting of dizziness, lightheadedness, and syncope.

Ventricular fibrillation

Ventricular fibrillation is usually fatal unless quickly rectified. Cerebral ischaemia occurs within 20 seconds, and irreversible brain damage at 3 minutes. Occasionally it is self-limiting. Treatment is a blow to precordium, DC shock (200 Joules), intravenous lignocaine, repeat DC shock if necessary, and intravenous betylium tosylate for recurring VF.

Sudden death (SD)

Sudden death is usually caused by ventricular fibrillation associated with coronary artery disease or, less frequently, cardiomyopathies. In 5–10% of survivors no cause is found.

Brugada syndrome

Brugada syndrome is associated with a family history of sudden death and is most prevalent in South-East Asia and Japan. The characteristic ECG abnormality is a right bundle branch pattern with ST elevation in leads V1–V3, occasionally with left axis deviation. Drug treatment is not beneficial. An implantable defibrillator is the best option at present.

Treatment of ventricular tachycardia

Acute

An intravenous lignocaine bolus (50–100 mg) should be followed by an intravenous infusion (procainamide is a valid option). DC shock should be administered if the patient is haemodynamically compromised (BP below 80 mmHg systolic). Intravenous amiodarone is given into a central vein, but the effect may take several hours.

Chronic

Beta-blockers should be given for non-sustained VT. Sotalol, mexiletine, disopyramide, amiodarone and implantable cardiac defibrillators are other options.

Additional notes

Electrophysiological study (EPS)

This is an invasive procedure undertaken under local anaesthesia. Several electrode catheters are introduced from a femoral vein, and normally from a femoral artery into the heart using complex ECG apparatus.

'Mapping' of abnormal conduction pathways are obtained. Stimulation of the heart is achieved through pacing wires to reproduce arrhythmias.

This can give clues to which medication might be appropriate in the treatment of a particular arrhythmia.

EPS is a prerequisite prior to ablation treatment.

Sinus node recovery time (overdrive suppression test)

This is used to assess the normality of the sinus-atrial node. The sensitivity of the test is not very satisfactory.

Historical notes

P Brugada, Spanish cardiologist, Heart Institute, Aalst, Belgium.

NJ Holter (1914–1983) USA. Provided technology for continuous ECG monitoring known as Holter monitor.

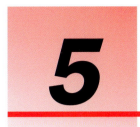

Hypertrophy

Left ventricular hypertrophy (LVH)

Increased voltages are detected over left ventricular leads.

A   Limb leads. When the R waves in lead I plus the S wave in lead III measure over 25 mm. When the R wave in aVL is over 11 mm or over 20 mm in aVF. Also when the S wave in aVR is greater than 14 mm.

B   Precordial leads. When the R wave in leads V5 or V6 plus the S wave in V1 measure over 35 mm. When the tallest R wave plus the tallest S wave measure over 45 mm, or when the R wave in V5 or V6 is greater than 26 mm.

Q waves in leads V1–V3 can indicate septal hypertrophy. LVH with strain has the same ECG appearance as LVH, with additional ST depression and T wave inversions in leads V4–V6 caused by underlying subendocardial ischaemia (ECGs 256–260).

Note that thin people with normal hearts can have increased voltages.

Causes of LVH

Hypertension, aortic valve disease, mitral incompetence, hypertrophic cardiomyopathy, and coarctation.

Right ventricular hypertrophy

Dominant R waves are seen in leads V1–V3 with T wave inversion (constituting RV strain). There is right axis deviation over 110° provided the QRS complex is under 120 milliseconds.

Causes of right ventricular hypertrophy

Pulmonary hypertension, pulmonary stenosis, Eisenmenger syndrome, acute pulmonary embolism and cor pulmonale.

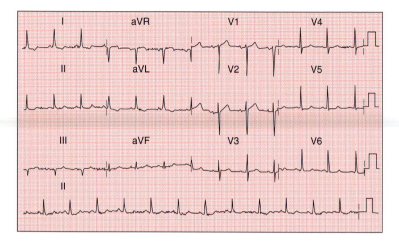

ECG 256: ECG from an elderly woman with moderate aortic stenosis (GT; 28/8/90).

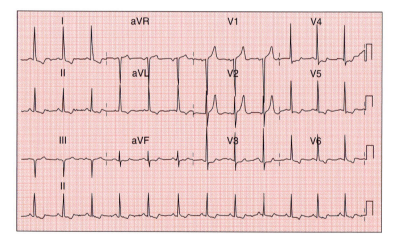

ECG 257: Seven years later there is severe aortic stenosis with left ventricular voltages and strain pattern. The patient had her aortic valve replaced (GT; 18/6/97).

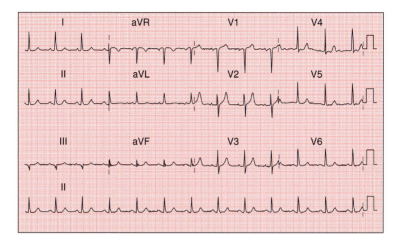

ECG 258: *Almost 2 years later the ECG appears remarkably normal. Biphasic P waves in lead V1 indicate residual left atrial hypertrophy (GT; 4/5/99).*

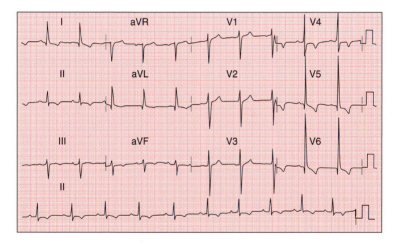

ECG 259: *ECG from a patient with severe aortic regurgitation showing LVH/strain pattern (HR; 10/2/88).*

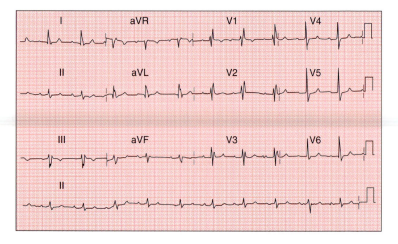

ECG 260: *There is marked improvement of the previous ECG changes 11 years later, after a successful aortic valve replacement. The patient has now developed right bundle branch with a prolonged PR interval (HR; 13/7/99).*

Left atrial hypertrophy

Wide notched P waves are seen in lead II. When these reach more than 120 milliseconds, the ECG is said to show 'P mitrale' (ECG 261). Biphasic P waves in lead V1 also indicate LAH (ECGs 262–268).

Causes of left atrial hypertrophy

Causes include increased left ventricular end diastolic pressure, ischaemic heart disease, hypertension, aortic and mitral valve disease and congenital shunting.

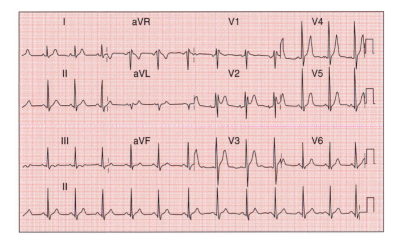

ECG 261: *ECG from a young patient with mild to moderate mitral stenosis showing P mitrale in lead II and biphasic P waves in lead V1 (MK; 17/3/99).*

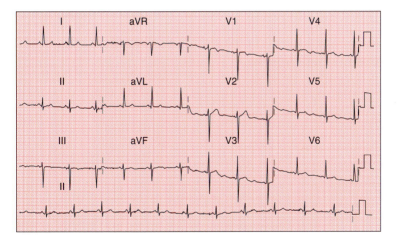

ECG 262: *Fairly normal electrocardiogram in an elderly woman with moderate aortic stenosis (JS; 21/11/95).*

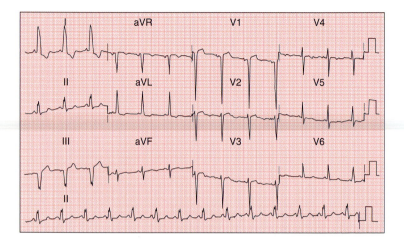

ECG 263: *Three years later there is left bundle branch block with left ventricular voltages and left atrial hypertrophy (biphasic P waves in lead V1). The patient now has severe aortic stenosis (JS; 10/7/98).*

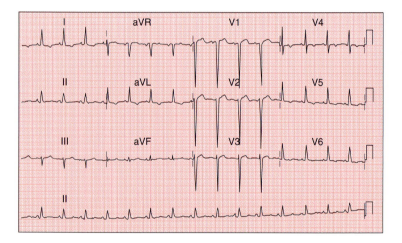

ECG 264: *Several weeks after aortic valve replacement, only left ventricular voltages and postoperative T wave inversions are visible (JS; 11/9/98).*

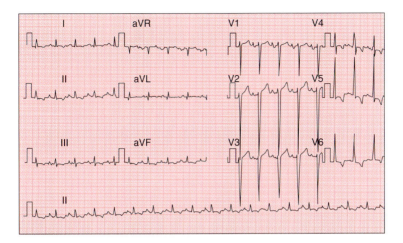

ECG 265: *Marked left atrial hypertrophy (biphasic P waves in lead V1) with LVH/strain pattern (HD; 27/3/95).*

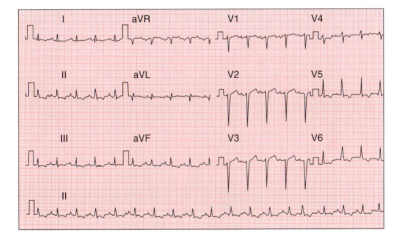

ECG 266: *Half-calibrated ECG from the same patient (precordial leads). The changes are much less evident. Always check calibration (HD; 27/3/95).*

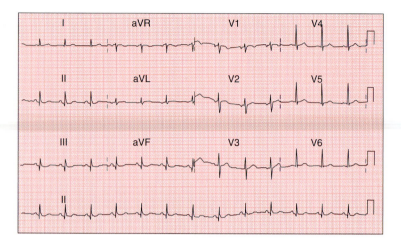

ECG 267: *Preoperative ECG prior to bypass surgery. The patient has been complaining of breathlessness. There are negative P waves in leads V1 and V2, indicating left atrial hypertrophy (HC; 10/10/97).*

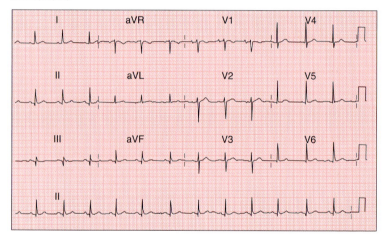

ECG 268: *Almost 2 years later the patient is much improved after bypass surgery. He no longer sufferes from breathlessness and the P waves in leads V1 and V2 have returned to normal (HC; 22/11/99).*

Right atrial hypertrophy

There are tall P waves present in leads II and V1. When these reach more than 2.5 mm (in lead II), the ECG is said to show 'P pulmonale'.

Causes of right atrial hypertrophy

Tricuspid and pulmonary valve disease, right heart failure, pulmonary embolism, right ventricular infarction and cor pulmonale.

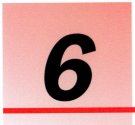

6 Cardiomyopathies and autoimmune disorders

Cardiomyopathy is defined as a disease of the myocardium without associated other recognisable pathologies.

Primary cardiomyopathies

There are three groups of primary cardiomyopathies:
- hypertrophic;
- dilated;
- restricted.

Hypertrophic (obstructive) cardiomyopathy (HOCM)

This inherited disorder is characterised by septal or apical hypertrophy and muscle cell disarray. The term obstructive refers to a left ventricular outflow tract gradient which is not invariably present.

ECG findings are as follows:
- LAD in 10-30% of cases;
- LVH in 50-75% of cases;
- precordial Q waves in leads V1-V3 are common;
- giant T wave inversions are common;
- SVT arrhythmia/AF are not infrequent;
- VT and AV block can occur, all badly tolerated owing to 'stiffness' of the left ventricle.

These are illustrated in ECGs 269-275.

Sudden death can occur, usually in young athletes. Right ventricular HOCM is rare.

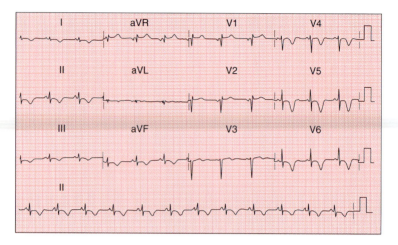

ECG 269: ECG from a middle-aged patient with classical hypertrophic cardiomyopathy. Note signs of left atrial hypertrophy in lead V1 and pronounced lateral T wave inversions (SS; 14/5/93).

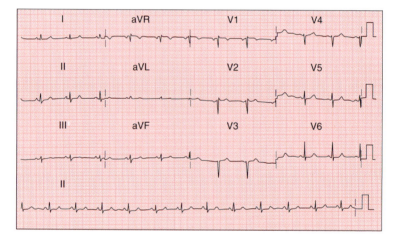

ECG 270: One year later the patient is on medication and remarkable improvement is seen in ECG indices. Left atrial hypertrophy remains. These pronounced T wave changes in hypertrophic cardiomyopathy can come and go, can be very confusing and lead to erroneous diagnosing of coronary artery disease (SS; 4/3/94).

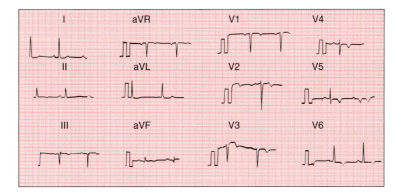

ECG 271: *Precordial T wave changes are present in this ECG from a patient with documented hypertrophic cardiomyopathy (SS; 4/1/95).*

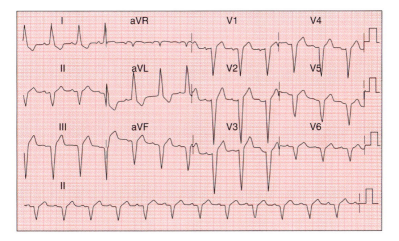

ECG 272: *Four years later, the patient has developed left bundle branch block (SS; 9/7/99).*

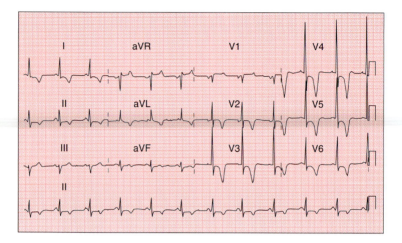

ECG 273: Hypertrophic cardiomyopathy. Very abnormal downward-pointing T waves with increased left ventricular voltages. Note also LAH (MR; 19/8/98).

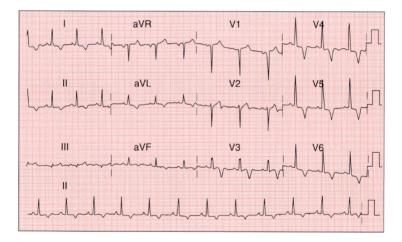

ECG 274: Another example of a patient with hypertrophic cardiomyopathy. The T wave inversions are often wrongly attributed to coronary artery disease. In fact the coronary arteries in hypertrophic cardiomyopathy are usually of large calibre and free from disease (PP; 20/7/98).

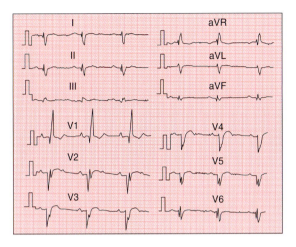

ECG 275: *Hypertrophic cardiomyopathy with normal coronary arteries. Septal Q waves are indicative of left ventricular hypertrophy. Right ventricular involvement is indicated by development of right axis deviation and right bundle branch block (WH; 7/8/97).*

Dilated cardiomyopathy

Dilated cardiomyopathy is characterised by an enlarged ventricle. ECG findings are listed below:

- LAH (notched P waves) is frequent;
- LVH in 30%;
- small QRS complexes if marked fibrotic changes affect the ventricles;
- LBBB is common;
- ST/T wave changes are common;
- AF and VPBs are common;
- VT–VF–SD are seen at the end stage of the disease.

These are illustrated in ECGs 276–279.

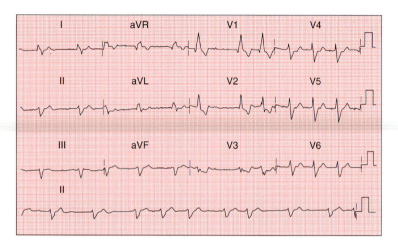

ECG 276: *Dilated cardiomyopathy in a renal failure patient receiving dialysis. There is atrial fibrillation, right bundle branch block and left axis deviation (GU; 27/11/98).*

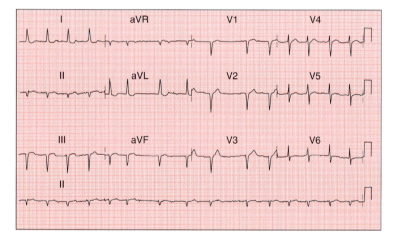

ECG 277: *This patient had a dilated cardiomyopathy and a normal coronary arteriogram. Note the inferior and anteroseptal Q waves. Atrial fibrillation is present (ES; 18/2/98).*

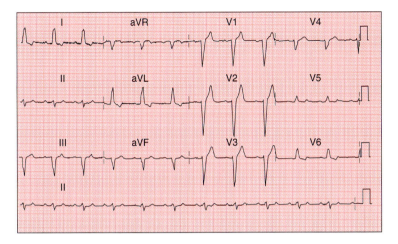

ECG 278: *Alcoholic dilated cardiomyopathy. There is left bundle branch block, left axis deviation and inferior Q waves (JB; 27/7/95).*

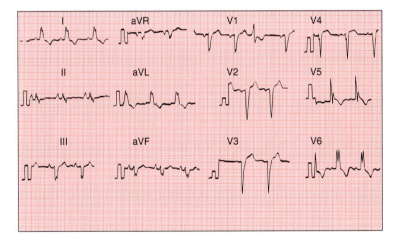

ECG 279: *Ischaemic cardiomyopathy caused by advanced coronary artery disease. There is left bundle branch block and marked left and right (V1–V2) atrial hypertrophy. P pulmonale in lead II denotes right atrial hypertrophy (AH; 13/9/95).*

Restrictive cardiomyopathy

Restrictive cardiomyopathy is the result of infiltration of the myocardium (for example in amyloid, haemochromatosis or fibrosis). There are no specific ECG changes.

Secondary cardiomyopathies

Duchenne muscular dystrophy

Tall R waves are seen in lead V1, and there is right bundle branch block and deep narrow Q waves.

Friedreich's ataxia

ST/T wave changes are common. Right axis deviation is more frequent than left. Tall R waves are seen in leads V1–V2. A short PR interval occurs in 25% of cases.

Myotonic dystrophy

Conduction defects are common.

Myxoedema

Characteristic ECG changes include small voltages, sinus bradycardia, and T wave changes.

Sarcoidosis

ECG changes include conduction defects (AV block), ectopic beats, and Q waves. There are no electrical signals from infiltrated areas (ECG 280).

Amyloid

There are low voltages, left axis deviation, conduction and rhythm defects. The disease can involve the coronary arteries, giving rise to infarction.

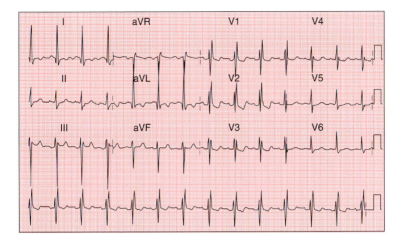

ECG 280: *Sarcoidosis with normal coronary arteries. Q waves are noted in leads I and aVL with T wave inversions and right bundle branch block (TD; 5/10/95).*

Autoimmune disorders

Scleroderma

Right ventricular hypertrophy is common (caused by pulmonary hypertension from lung involvement). Left ventricular hypertrophy can occur if the renal arteries are involved.

Systemic lupus erythematosis (SLE) and polyarteritis nodosa (PAN)

T wave changes, caused by pericarditis, are seen. Vasculitis can give rise to myocardial infarction.

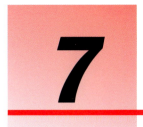

7

Pericarditis, myocarditis and metabolic disorders

Pericarditis

Acute

Acute pericarditis is characterised by ST elevation (concave upward) in leads facing the effusion (ECGs 281–283). Usually there are widespread T wave inversions. In addition, the ECG can exhibit P wave changes, low voltage QRS complexes arrhythmias and electrical alternans (alternating size of P, QRS and T waves [ECG 284]). Lead aVR shows ST segment depression (reflecting heart cavity signals).

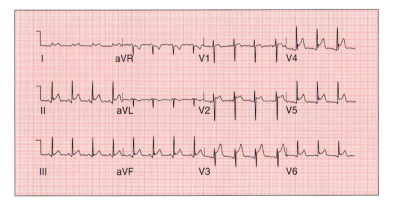

ECG 281: *ECG showing classical changes of pericardial effusion (concave ST elevation). This 23-year-old man had attempted suicide with a nail gun to the anterior chest wall. Courtesy of Dr DH Spodick. Previously published Clin Cardiol 1999;* **22**: *544.*

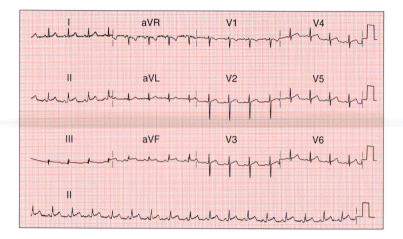

ECG 282: This black patient presented with documented tuberculous pericarditis during pregnancy. Note the ST elevation, particularly in leads II, III and aVF, and less so in leads V4–V6 (Mrs M; 9/10/92).

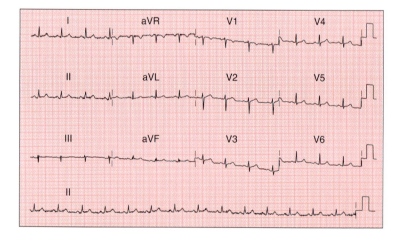

ECG 283: Three years later, after tapping and treating, the ST elevations have disappeared (Mrs M; 3/4/95).

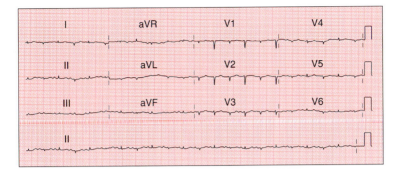

ECG 284: *This is a good example of electrical alternans, which is particularly well seen in leads V1 and V2. (FO; April 1997).*

Chronic

Chronic pericarditis produces small voltages, T wave inversions, arrhythmias, abnormal P waves and right axis deviation (ECG 285). Similar changes are seen in hypothyroidism, hypopituitism, obesity and emphysema.

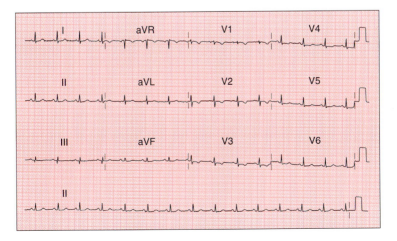

ECG 285: *Chronic non-specific benign pericarditis. The patient had a normal coronary arteriogram. The ECG shows T wave and ST changes in the precordial leads (DS; 10/7/98).*

Myocarditis

Viral

ST/T wave changes and AV block are not uncommon (ECGs 286 and 287). Occasionally there are Q waves, mimicking acute myocardial infarction.

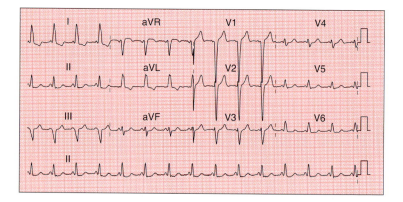

ECG 286: *This middle-aged woman was diagnosed with acute viral myocarditis. She presented with sudden onset left ventricular failure. The ECG shows left bundle branch block (FO; 8/4/97).*

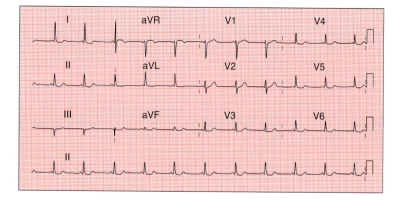

ECG 287: *The patient improved greatly with medication and the ECG changes returned to normal (FO; 9/7/97).*

Rheumatic fever

First degree heart block is common with a prolonged PR interval. ST/T wave changes are often present. Junctional rhythm can develop.

AIDS

AIDS-related myocarditis produces ST/T wave changes and bundle branch block on the ECG.

Chagas' disease

T wave changes are seen with right bundle branch block and ventricular premature beats (VPBs).

Drugs, electrolytes and metabolic disturbances

Drugs

Digoxin

Digoxin causes ST depression with small T waves that are biphasic and negative. There is a short QT interval, with an increase in size of U waves. In addition, it can cause arrhythmias, ventricular premature beats and junctional rhythms. There may be AV dissocation, AV block, sinoatrial dysfunction or supraventricular arrhythmias (atrial tachycardia). An example of digoxin toxicity is illustrated in ECGs 288–290.

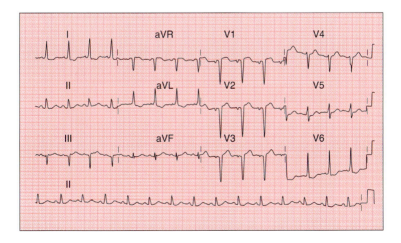

ECG 288: *This elderly woman with renal and heart failure and moderate aortic stenosis has incomplete left bundle branch block. There are ST changes in leads I, aVL and V6, and left atrial hypertrophy (LB; 10/4/95).*

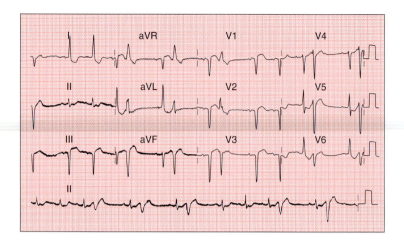

ECG 289: *Same patient with digoxin toxicity (digoxin, toxic level 3.4). There are marked ST segment changes in leads I and aVL, along with ventricular extrasystoles (LB; 22/4/95).*

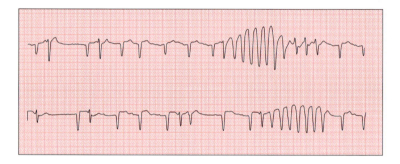

ECG 290: *The patient's condition worsened as she developed ventricular tachycardia and ventricular fibrillation. She died despite medication (LB; 23/4/95).*

Quinidine

Quinidine produces small inverted T waves, ST depression, increased U waves and a prolonged QT interval. Similar changes are seen with disopyramide and procainamide.

Phenothiazine and tricyclic antidepressants

These drugs produce ECG changes similar to those caused by quinidine.

Lithium

Lithium causes T wave changes and sinoatrial disorders (for example sinus bradycardia and SA block).

Cocaine

Cocaine causes coronary spasm (marked by transient ST elevation) and myocardial infarction (Q and non Q wave). Ventricular tachycardia and ventricular fibrillation can occur.

Electrolytes and metabolic disturbances

Hypokalaemia

ECG changes include arrhythmias and AV block, ST depression, large R waves, wide QRS complexes and P wave changes.

Hyperkalaemia

In hyperkalaemia, the ECG will inscribe arrhythmias (bradycardia/tachycardia, or AV block), peaked T waves, small or absent P waves, wide, bizarre QRS complexes and ST elevation.

Hypercalcaemia

Hypercalcaemia produces a shortened QT interval.

Hypocalcaemia

Hypocalcaemia produces a prolonged QT interval.

Hypermagnesaemia

In hypermagnesaemia there are prolonged PR intervals and QRS complexes. AV block can also occur.

Hypomagnesaemia

There are narrow QRS complexes, peaked T waves and prominent U waves.

Altered sodium concentration

Changes in sodium concentration do not produce specific ECG changes.

Hypothermia

In hypothermia, the ECG shows sinus bradycardia. There are prolonged PR and QT intervals. J waves (a signal between QRS and ST segments) are present.

8

Pacemakers, ICDs (implantable cardiac defibrillators) and cardioversion

Pacemakers

Pacemakers were first introduced in 1958 by Senning as a treatment for complete heart block. They now have much wider applications. The system consists of a battery operated generator (pacemaker) and electrodes (leads) which stimulate the heart. Pacemakers are inserted under local anaesthesia. The electrode is placed into the right ventricle and or right atrium, either by cutting down on a cephalic vein or by subclavian Seldinger technique. The position of the electrode is checked radiologically. Electronic parameters are obtained and need to be entirely satisfactory. A subcutaneous pocket is then created to position the generator. Very rarely, when venous systems prove inadequate, an epicardial approach is required, using a corkscrew electrode, through a small thoracotomy. The tip of the electrode (which makes contact with the myocardium) can be unipolar or bipolar.

Pacemakers are affected by high powered electromagnetic environments such as radar installations, microwave ovens, certain cordless telephones and security screening at airports. Patients have to be warned about these hazards. Detailed international identity cards are provided and should be carried at all times.

Permanent pacemakers

Unipolar leads are prone to extrinsic electrical signals which can inhibit the ventricular output (myopotential interference). Bipolar leads are now preferred.

Nomenclature

Four letters conventionally describe the pacing mode.

1st letter: **Chamber paced**

V = ventricle

A = atrium

D = dual chamber (atrium and ventricle)

2nd letter: **Chamber sensed**

V = ventricle

A = atrium

D = dual chamber

3rd letter: **Mode of response**

I = inhibited output

T = triggered output

D = both inhibited and triggered

0 = none

4th letter: **Programmability**

P = simple programmable

M = multiprogrammable

R = rate variation in response to a sensed variable

The latter permits an increase in pacing rate. Different types of sensors are stimulated by physical exertion according to the patient's demands and the generator is activated accordingly.

Indications for permanent pacing

Symptomatic bradycardias

Permanent pacing is indicated for sinoatrial disease, slow atrial fibrillation (prolonged pauses lasting over 3 seconds), AV block, second degree or complete heart block (Adams–Stokes attacks), symptomatic fascicular block (bi- and trifascicular), and carotid sinus syndrome with pauses of 3 seconds or more on carotid massage.

Asymptomatic bradycardias

A heart rate below 40 beats per minute, periods of asystole and atrial fibrillation/flutter with pauses over 3 seconds will benefit from pacemaker implantation.

Tilt test causing profound bradycardia

The test is undertaken to ascertain a patient's response to tilting at 60% for 45 minutes. Special attention is given to detect a drop in heart rate and in blood pressure. It is a test of autonomous nervous system integrity.

Other indications

Some patients with hypertrophic obstructive cardiomyopathy, dilated cardiomyopathy and intractable congestive cardiac failure will benefit from dual chamber pacing. Haemodynamic improvement can result from careful programming of the AV sequential interval.

Pacemaker syndrome

This refers to symptoms attributed to a fall in systolic pressure resulting from loss of AV synchrony, atrial contraction against a closed tricuspid valve and retrograde P activation. This is seen with VVI systems. Symptoms of syncope, dizziness and fatigue, can be remedied by upgrading the patient to a dual chamber system.

Types of pacemakers in use

VVI	One lead to the right ventricle.
DDD	One lead to the right atrium, and one to the right ventricle.
VDD	One lead to the right ventricle with a sensor in the right atrium (all on one lead).
AAI	Atrial pacing mainly for sick sinus syndrome.
AV Sequential	Pacing the right atrium and right ventricle, thus adding atrial contribution to the overall cardiac output (DDD-VDD). This is physiologically superior, but cannot be used in atrial fibrillation.
Biventricular	One lead to the right ventricle, one lead to the coronary sinus. Presently being evaluated for improving left ventricular function in severely compromised patients.

ECGs 291–312 were recorded from patients with various types of pacemaker.

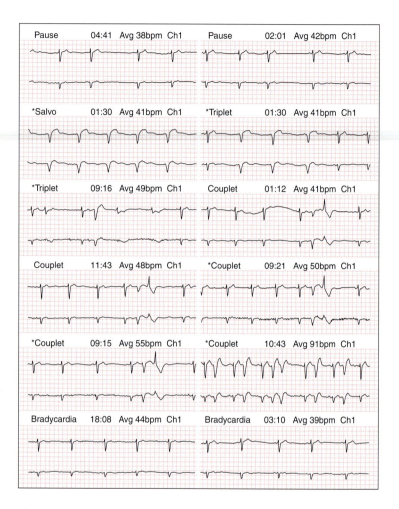

ECG 291: *This middle-aged patient with numerous TIAs was diagnosed suffering from sick sinus syndrome. The upper trace shows evidence of sinoatrial disease. There are episodes of atrial fibrillation lower down the recording (Mr M; 1995).*

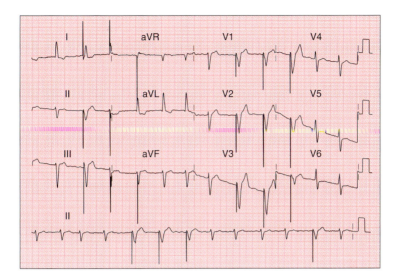

ECG 292: *The patient had a VVI pacemaker. This trace shows demand pacing activity with underlying atrial fibrillation. No further TIAs were reported (Mr M; 27/3/95).*

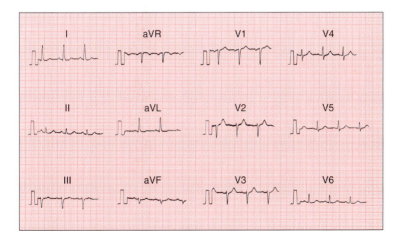

ECG 293: *Normal electrocardiogram from an elderly woman (WP; 28/9/93).*

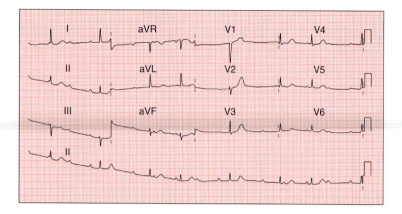

ECG 294: *The same patient, 5 years later, has complete heart block. The ventricular rate is 40 beats per minute and there are narrow QRS complexes. The P rate is about 90 beats per minute (WP; 26/11/98).*

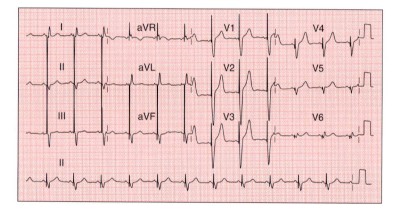

ECG 295: *After insertion of a VDD pacemaker, each P wave is followed by a pacing signal. The single electrode has a sensing device 'floating' in the right atrium which picks up atrial activity and then transmits a signal to the ventricles so that AV sequential activation is maintained (WP; 27/11/98).*

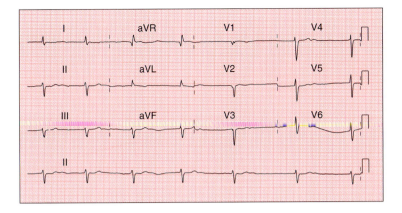

ECG 296: *Complete heart block with underlying atrial fibrillation. The ventricular rate is 39 beats per minute (AJ; 19/1/99).*

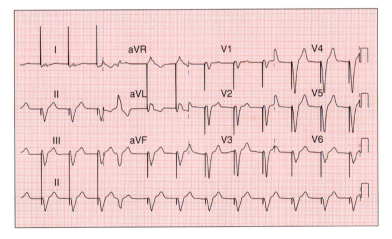

ECG 297: *After insertion of a VVI pacemaker, the ventricular rate is 67 beats per minute. There is no AV sequential pacing in this case. Retrograde P waves are seen in lead I (AJ; 22/1/99).*

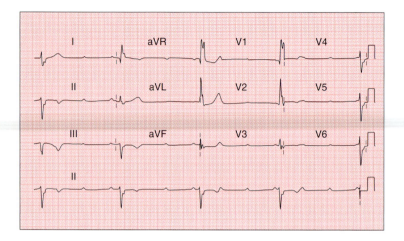

ECG 298: *Complete heart block. There is AV dissociation, wide QRS complexes, and a ventricular rate of 25 beats per minute (GM; 7/3/99).*

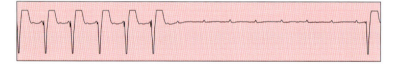

ECG 299: *Rhythm strip from the same patient showing good pacing activity to the left. P waves are only seen to the right of the strip. The patient is completely dependent on pacing as demonstrated during pacemaker check (GM; March 1999).*

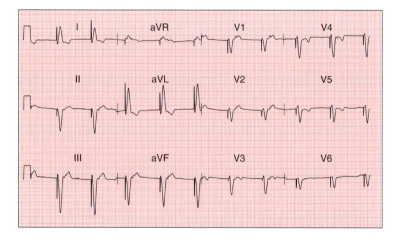

ECG 300: *VVI pacing showing retrograde P waves. The patient is well, with no symptoms (PD; 16/8/99).*

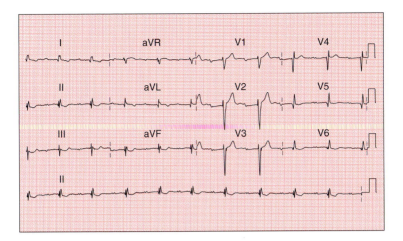

ECG 301: *A 72-year-old patient who had undergone bypass surgery years before, was diagnosed with first degree heart block (WN; 10/5/99).*

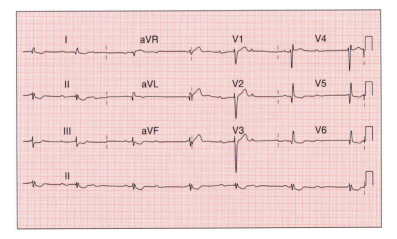

ECG 302: *The same patient, several days later, progressed to complete heart block; best seen in rhythm strip (lead IV) (WN; 28/5/99).*

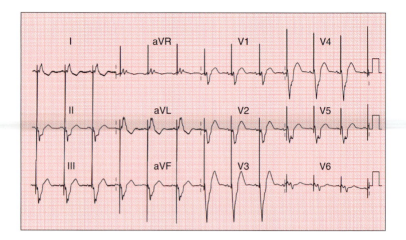

ECG 303: *After insertion of a VDD pacemaker there was a good AV sequential response (WN; 12/6/99).*

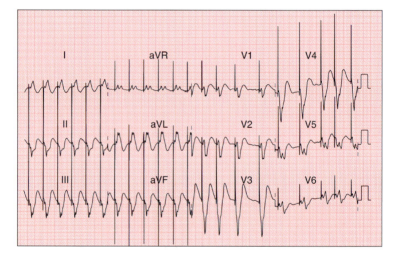

ECG 304: *The patient suddenly felt unwell; his blood pressure dropped to 90/47 mmHg with signs of tachycardia. This was attributed to improper setting of the pacemaker which is sensing inappropriately. The pacemaker was reset and all was well (WN; 12/6/99).*

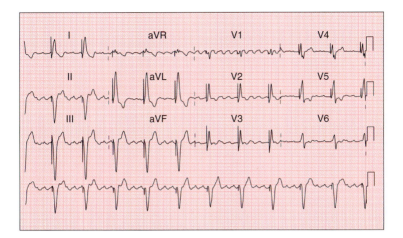

ECG 305: *Pacing activity with underlying atrial flutter. The P rate is 300 beats per minute (GB; 16/12/98).*

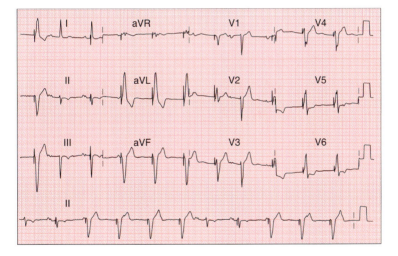

ECG 306: *The same patient has underlying complete heart block. Dissociated P waves are clearly seen in lead V1 (GB; 1999).*

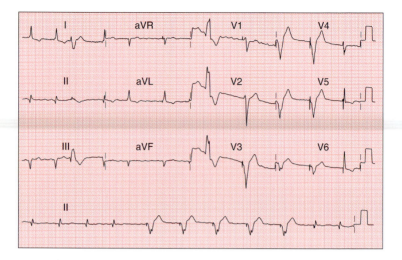

ECG 307: *ECG from a patient who had undergone two bypass operations and had poor LV function. A VVI pacemaker was inserted for episodic slow atrial fibrillation. The rhythm strip clearly shows atrial fibrillation and pacey activity (PP; 2/10/98).*

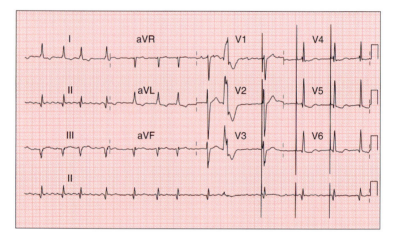

ECG 308: *Several weeks later the rhythm strip at the bottom shows that pacing is not capturing well. The middle of the three pacing beats shows a prolonged pacing to the QRS interval which is also seen in leads V4, V5 and V6. This resulted from dislodgement of the pace wire (PP; 23/11/98).*

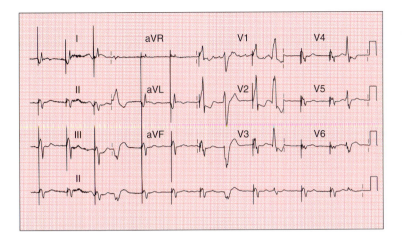

ECG 309: *The patient then had a biventricular system inserted (for reduced LV function). One electrode was placed in the right ventricle and the other in the coronary sinus. Two clear pacing signals are seen in leads V4, V5 and V6 (PP; 12/5/99).*

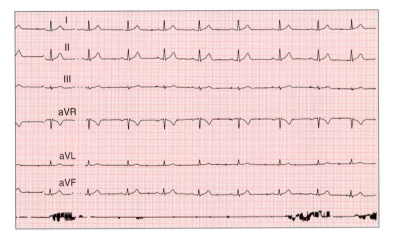

ECG 310: *Beginning of a tilt test in a 40-year-old librarian who was suffering from syncopal attacks (KD; September 1999).*

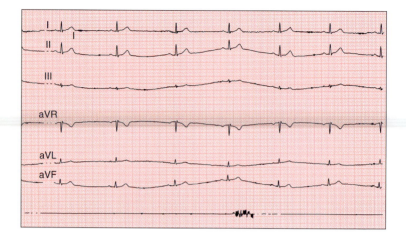

ECG 311: *The patient's heart rate dropped, down to 20 beats per minute, as he fainted during the tilt test (KD; September 1999).*

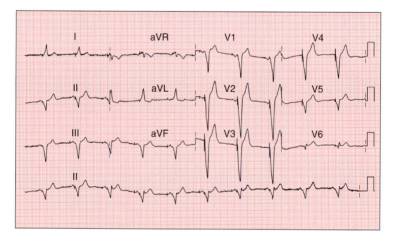

ECG 312: *A dual chamber pacemaker was inserted. The two pacing signals are seen clearly in the rhythm strip at the bottom, stimulating first the atria and then the ventricles in sequence. No further symptoms were reported (KD; 15/9/99).*

Myopotential inhibition

The generator senses pectoral muscle activity and ceases to function temporarily (seen with unipolar leads).

Hysteresis

This consists of programming the 'escape interval' to be longer than the pacing interval. The patient's sinus rhythm can function at a lower rate than the pacing rate (sinus rhythm is more physiological than VVI pacing).

Follow up

Follow up is undertaken in specialised pacing clinics. Modern generators are interrogated and programmed non-invasively. Battery depletion can now be predicted fairly accurately.

Failure to pace

This is uncommon nowadays but can occur as a result of any of the following:

- migration of electrodes (particularly in the first few days after implantation only);
- high threshold (exit block), for example thrombus formation at tip of electrode; or fibrotic changes in a damaged right ventricle;
- damaged electrodes (occasional perforation of myocardium);
- faulty generator (very rare nowadays).

Complications of pacemakers

Complications are rare but can include:

- infection;
- thrombosis of the vein in which the pace wire is inserted;
- perforation of the myocardium;
- tamponade.

Temporary pacing

An electrode is inserted into the right ventricle (through the femoral vein, external jugular, subclavian or brachial vein) and is connected to a non-implanted generator.

Indications

Indications include second or third degree heart block particularly after myocardial infarction. Preoperatively, it can be used in the presence of important bradycardia and during angioplasty in selected cases. Permanent and temporary pacing are covered with antibiotic medication. It is customary to give a course for several days after implantation. Antibiotic powder can also be inserted into the subcutaneous pouch at the time of generator implantation.

Occasionally, pacing can be useful to correct a supraventricular or ventricular arrhythmia by a method known as 'overpacing'. The technique consists of pacing 'temporarily' at a rate above the arrhythmia and then bringing down the pace rate to reestablish sinus conduction.

External pacemakers

These fairly crude devices can be life-saving. They are unpleasant for the patient, consisting of large plate electrodes that are applied to the thorax in extreme situations, while awaiting proper pacemaker implantation. They are painful to the patient, who will need profound sedation.

General precautions

DC cardioversion is usually possible in patients with pacemakers. If in doubt, obtain the manufacturer's advice. The electrodes should be kept as far a possible from the pacemaker site. Mobile telephones can interfere with pacing activity and should be tested individually.

Implantable cardioverter/defibrillators (ICDs)

These devices sense the onset of a ventricular tachycardia or fibrillation and respond by sending out an electrical discharge to restore sinus rhythm. Low energy is used for cardioversion and high energy for defibrillation which can be fairly unpleasant for the patient. The system also acts as a pacemaker for bradycardias.

Initially external electrodes were applied around the heart, necessitating thoracotomy. The present models use transvenous electrodes and the generators are only slightly larger than an ordinary pacemaker.

Clinical trials have recently demonstrated that ICDs are superior to antiarrhythmic medication for VT/VF. Atrial defibrillators are presently being evaluated.

Driving

Patients fitted with permanent pacemakers and ICDs have to report to the national driving authority. Ordinary pacing allows continued driving. ICD regulations are more complex.

Cardioversion

Direct current (DC) cardioversion is the delivery of an electrical shock to the heart to depolarise the myocardium. This allows the sinus node to regain control. The procedure requires a short acting general anaesthesia.

Internal defibrillators

Internal defibrillators are used during open heart surgery. The electrodes are placed directly over the myocardium.

External defibrillators

Two electrodes are applied to the chest, each electrode is marked sternum or apex. The skin is covered with a gel pad (to prevent burning). The patient is heavily sedated or given a short anaesthetic for elective procedures. The energy delivered is measured in Joules. Atrial flutter requires 50 Joules, while atrial fibrillation and VT/VF usually require a starting at 200 Joules, building up to 360 Joules if necessary. Synchronisation is used to avoid discharging on the patient's T wave, which could induce ventricular arrhythmias (ECG 205). As the shock is delivered all assisting personnel must not touch the patient.

Risks

Cardioversion can cause occasional profound bradycardia requiring intravenous atropine or even temporary pacing.

Systemic emboli at the time of cardioversion or in weeks following the event have been known to occur. It is therefore essential that the patient is given adequate anticoagulation. In established cases warfarin is the drug of choice; the INR should be between 2.0 and 2.5. In acute cases, a bolus of intravenous heparin (5000 units half an hour before cardioversion) is indicated.

It has been shown that amiodarone given for a few weeks prior to, or atropine at the time, of DC conversion will improve the success rate. After successful DC conversion, recurrence of the arrhythmia can be prevented by the use of flecainide, propafenone, sotalol or amiodarone. Quinidine is still in use in the United States.

Emergency cardioversion

For VT/VF, immediate DC shock is indicated without synchronisation. The procedure is usually supplemented by intravenous lignocaine or bretylium tosylate, particularly in resistant ventricular arrhythmias. Cardiopulmonary resuscitation (CPR) may be required.

For uncontrolled supraventricular tachycardia with cardiogenic shock (BP below 80 mmHg systolic), synchronisation is applied and intravenous heparin and sedation are indicated.

Historical notes

A Senning (1915–2000) Swedish professor of surgery, Zurich, Switzerland.

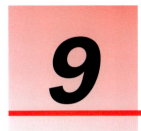

9

Mixed ECG quizzes

If you have read the previous pages you should now be able to interpret ECGs 313–350. The aim of the book is not to turn you into an expert, but to enable you to read basic electrocardiograms. This should give you a certain amount of satisfaction and at least prove beneficial to the patients under your care.

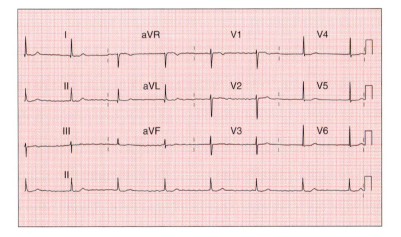

ECG 313: *Atrial fibrillation and complete heart block, hence the regularity of the trace. The ventricular rate is 43 beats per minute. This exemplifies a nodal escape mechanism (Mrs S; 30/12/99).*

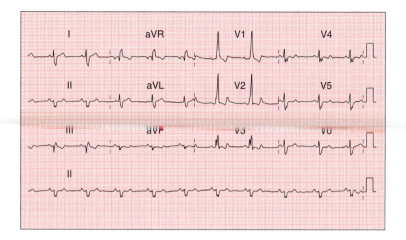

ECG 314: Right bundle branch block. Possible right ventricular hypertrophy (Mr B; 8/9/98).

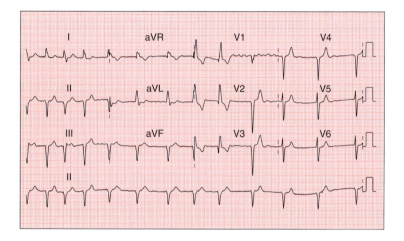

ECG 315: Atrial fibrillation, left axis deviation, right bundle branch block, anteroseptal and inferior Q waves. Probable inferior and anterior infarctions. (Bifascicular block.) (WF; 11/8/98).

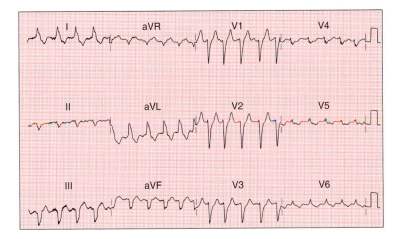

ECG 316: *Atrial fibrillation, left bundle branch block and reduced R waves over the precordium suggestive of anterolateral damage (AR; 24/9/95).*

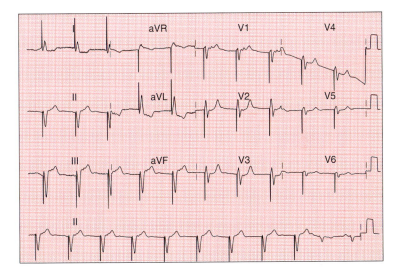

ECG 317: *VVI pacing. Retrograde P waves are seen in the bottom strip (AR; 26/9/95).*

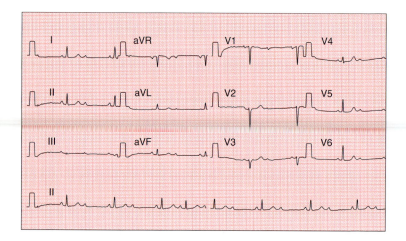

ECG 318: *2:1 AV block (Mobitz II). Second degree (BN; 7/2/97).*

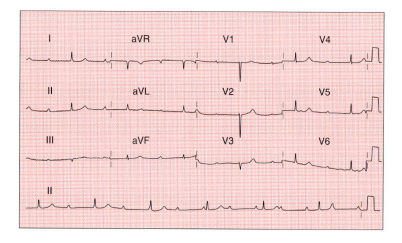

ECG 319: *Complete heart block (third degree). AV dissociation. The P rate exceeds the QRS rate (BN; 18/2/97).*

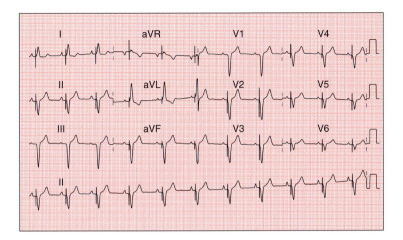

ECG 320: *VDD pacing (NB; 21/2/97).*

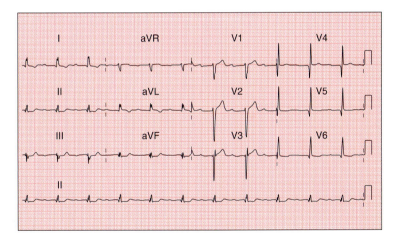

ECG 321: *First degree AV block with anterolateral Q waves (WN; 18/6/97).*

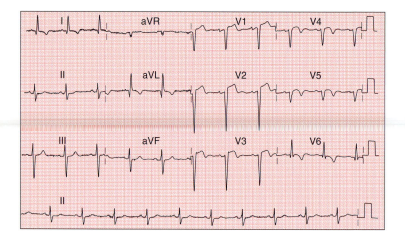

ECG 322: *Anteroseptal Q waves. Left ventricular aneurysm is indicated by marked ST elevation in leads V1 and V3 (HH; 18/11/91).*

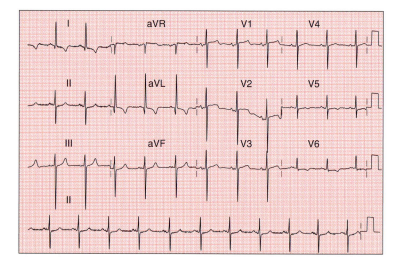

ECG 323: *Abnormal ECG. This patient had a normal coronary arteriogram. No cause was found for the ECG abnormality which would otherwise indicate coronary artery disease or some cardiomyopathy (ME; 6/4/94).*

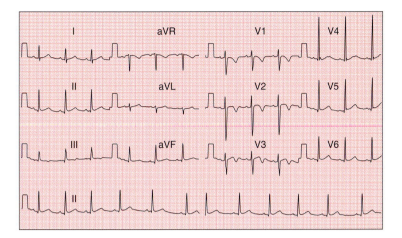

ECG 324: *'Athlete's Heart'. Well trained athletes develop ECG abnormalties that often lead to unnecessary investigations (PK; 26/2/96).*

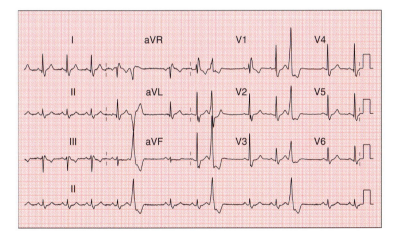

ECG 325: *Right bundle branch block. Unifocal ventricular extrasystoles (right bundle branch pattern originating from the left ventricle) (RL; 5/1/99).*

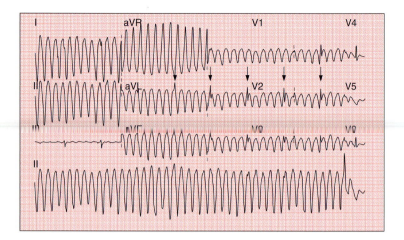

ECG 326: *Tremor giving the appearance of ventricular tachycardia. Courtesy Dr R Llinas and Dr GV Henderson. Previuously published in Images Clin Med 1999; **341**: 1275.*

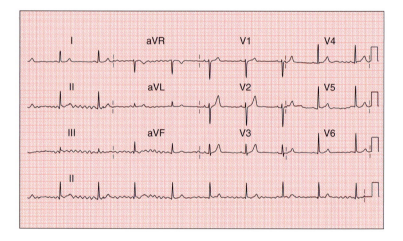

ECG 327: *Artefact, again due to tremor (Mr W; 20/10/99).*

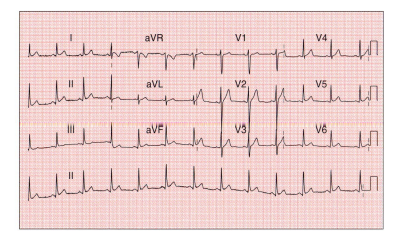

ECG 328: *'High uptake' giving rise to ST elevation. This is a normal finding in black patients. Note LV voltages (JL; 18/10/99).*

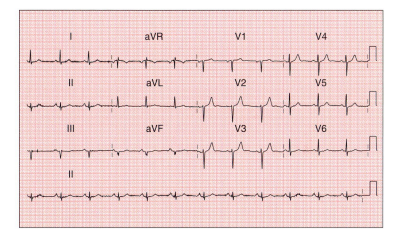

ECG 329: *Inferior Q waves obtained in a supine patient (PC; 18/10/99).*

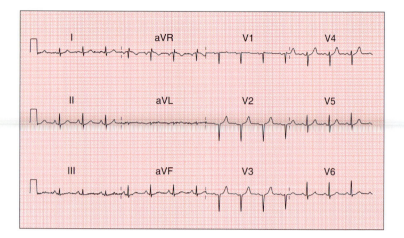

ECG 330: *ECG from the same patient, now standing. The Q waves have disappeared. They are 'positional' and not pathological (PC; 18/10/99).*

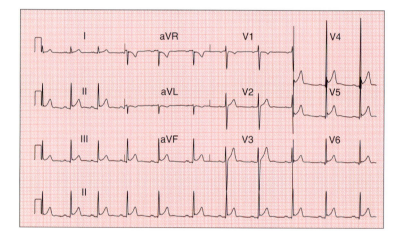

ECG 331: *High ST uptake in a black patient. Normal ECG (GN; 18/3/99).*

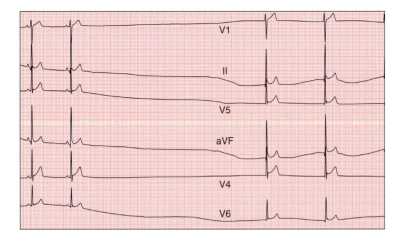

ECG 332: *Cardiac standstill. This 14-year-old boy with syncopal attacks had a positive tilt test. He was subsequently successfully paced (RS; 22/12/99).*

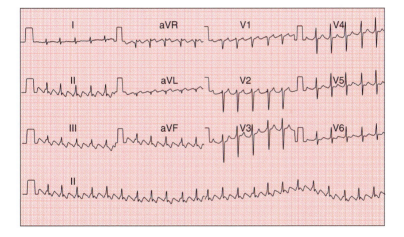

ECG 333: *Atrial flutter (EB; 6/12/96).*

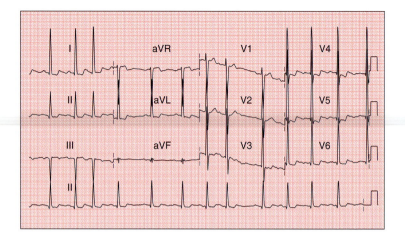

ECG 334: *Left ventricular hypertrophy/strain. Atrial extrasystoles (severe aortic regurgitation) (FM; 18/8/99).*

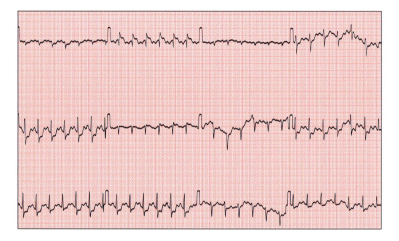

ECG 335: *Positive stress test. Marked ST ischaemic changes in inferolateral leads at heart rate of 150 beats per minute (EM; 19/11/93).*

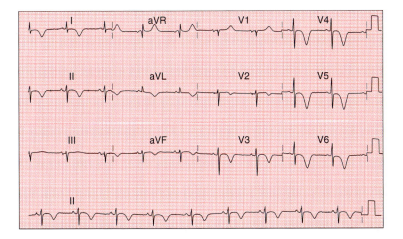

ECG 336: *Young woman with hypertrophic cardiomyopathy and normal coronary arteries. These marked T wave inversions were not seen 1 year later on medication (EM; 19/11/93).*

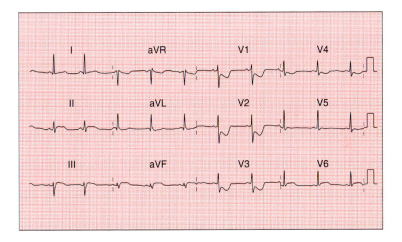

ECG 337: *Acute subendocardial infarction. Elderly Asian woman (Mrs H; 11/7/99).*

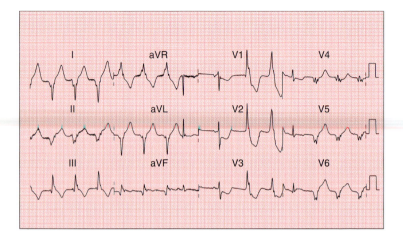

ECG 338: *Same patient developing slow ventricular tachycardia several hours later. This does not require treatment (Mrs H; 11/7/99).*

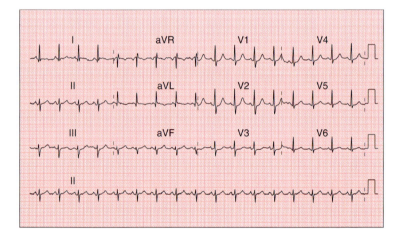

ECG 339: *Two days later with medication, marked improvement. Dominant R wave in V1 and V2 due to true posterior infarction (SP; 13/7/99).*

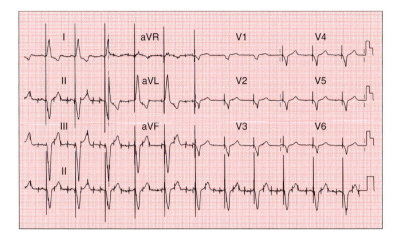

ECG 340: *Patient with VDD pacemaker. Abnormal vertical spikes are visible in the inferior leads. These were due to inappropriate electrode contact with left leg (SP; 15/3/00).*

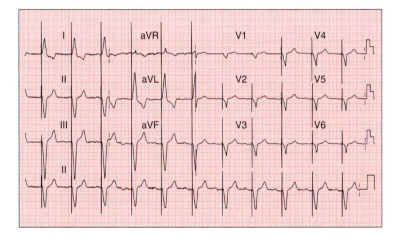

ECG 341: *Situation rectified. Proper application of electrodes is important. Dried electrodes will cause artefacts (SP; 15/3/00).*

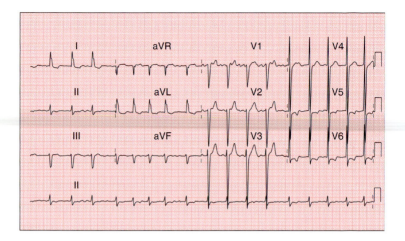

ECG 342: *Atrial fibrillation. Left ventricle hypertrophy/strain pattern widened QRS all due to severe hypertension (JW; 2/2/98).*

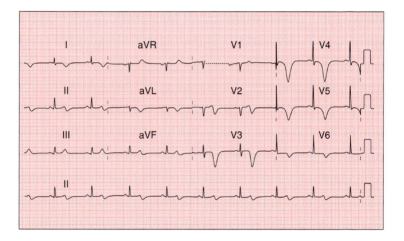

ECG 343: *Subendocardial infarction (AS; 28/12/95).*

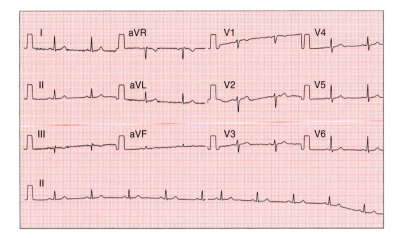

ECG 344: Four months later good resolution is seen (AS; 22/4/96).

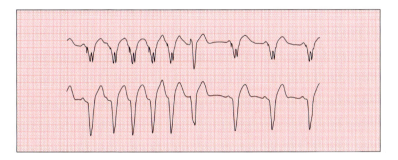

ECG 345: Pacemaker-induced tachycardia. The patient was aware of palpitation. There is inappropriate pacing due to incorrect sensing, giving rise to a reentry phenomenon. The situation is rectified by modifying the generator settings (LE; 1999).

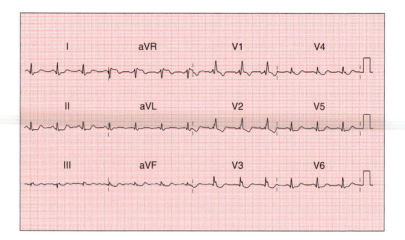

ECG 346: *Elderly woman with previous CABG. There is normal electric axis, right bundle branch block and small anterior Q waves (MB; 8/3/00).*

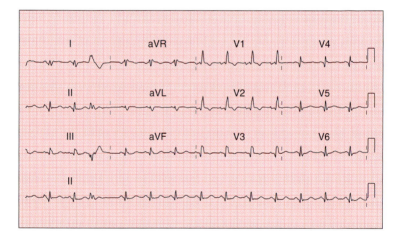

ECG 347: *Same woman a few days later with 'extension' of previous infarction. Q waves are now clearly seen in leads V2 to V6 and the axis has changed indicating posterior hemi block, the new infarction having involved the conducting system (MB; 13/3/00).*

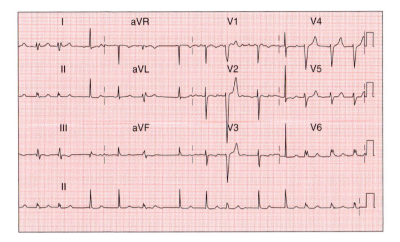

ECG 348: *There is AF with intermittent LBBB. This is rate dependent (aberration). The RR intervals of the LBBB complexes are slightly shorter than the narrow complexes. (RC; October 2000).*

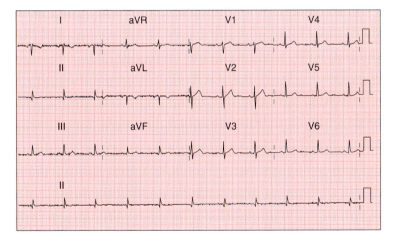

ECG 349: *Difficult ECG to interpret. This is due to inversion of the limb leads. This can be very confusing. (RV; October 2000).*

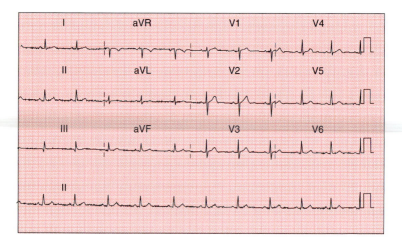

ECG 350: *Same as ECG 349, with electrodes properly connected. This is the author's ECG which he regards as normal. (RV; October 2000).*

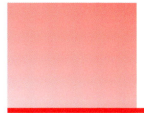

Further reading

Chapter 1

Shamroth L. An introduction to electrocardiography. Blackwell Scientific Publication. Oxford, 1971.

Chapter 2

Sclarowsky, S. Electrocardiography of acute myocardial ischaemic syndromes. Martin Dunitz. London, 1999.

Chapter 3

Macfarlane, PW. Renaissance in electrocardiography. *Lancet* 1999; 353: 1377–9.

Mangrum JM, DiMarco JP. The evaluation and management of bradycardia. *N Engl J Med* 2000; 342: 703–9.

Chapter 4

English KM, Channer KS. Managing atrial fibrillation in elderly people. *BMJ* 1999; 318: 1088–9.

Bennett DH. Cardiac arrhythmias. Butterworth Heinemann. Oxford, 1998.

Ganz LI, Friedman PL. Supraventricular tachycardia. *N Engl J Med* 1995; 332: 162–73.

Chapter 5

Chuan Chou TC. Electrocardiography in clinical practice (adult and paediatric). WB Saunders Co. Philadelphia, 1996.

Hirsch J, Wirtz JI. New antithrombolytic agents. *Lancet* 1999; 353: 1431–6.

Chapter 8

Morley-Davies A, Cobbe SM. Cardiac pacing. *Lancet* 1997; 349: 41–6.

Opie LH. Drugs for the heart. WB Saunders Co. Philadelphia, 1995.

Vlay, SC. A practical approach to cardiac arrhythmias. Little Brown & Co. Boston, 1996.

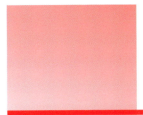

Drug regimen tables

Table 1: *Antiarrhythmic agents*

Name	Mode of action	Indications	Side effects
Class Ia	*Sodium channel blockers*	Atrial and ventricular arrhythmias	
Quinidine**	Prolong QT interval		Torsade de pointes
Disopyramide**			Hypotension, urinary retention, dry mouth
Procainamide**			Hypotension, haematological and SLE
Class Ib	Shorten QT interval	Ventricular arrhythmias	
Lignocaine†			CNS
Mexiletine†			CNS, bradycardia, hypotension
Tocainide†			CNS, haematological
Phenytoin†			Hypotension, CNS, gingivitis, SLE, pulmonary
Class Ic	No effect on QT	Atrial and ventricular arrhythmias (WPW)	
Flecainide**			Negative inotropism, pro-arrhythmic
Propafenone**			Similar to flecainide, mild beta-blocking property
Class II	*Beta-blockers*	Atrial and ventricular arrhythmias	
Beta-blockers*	Reduce sympathetic activity AV nodal slowing		Bronchospasm, claudication, bradycardia, cold extremeties
Class III	*Potassium channel blockers*		
Amiodarone**	Prolongs QT interval, long half life	Atrial and ventricular arrhythmias	Systemic side effects, skin, eyes, liver, lungs, thyroid
Sotalol			Beta-blocker and amiodarone properties, but not as toxic
Bretylium		Resistant VT/VF	Hypotension
Azimilide		Atrial fibrillation	
Class IV	*Calcium channel blockers*	Atrial arrhythmias (also right ventricular outflow and fasicular VT) Not used for sick sinus syndrome or WPW syndrome	
Verapamil*	Slow down SA and AV nodes		Severe bradycardia (if given with beta-blockers), negative inotropism, constipation
Diltiazem*			As verapamil. Generally milder, no constipation
Digitalis*	Increases vagal tone	Atrial fibrillation, atrial flutter, SVT, not WPW	Toxicity, anorexia, nausea, diarrhoea, proarrhythmic, visual
Adenosine	Powerful AV node blocker	Re-entrant SVT	Short-lived. Care with asthmatic and sick sinus syndrome
Atropine	Antivagal effect	Sinoatrial brady-cardia, asystole	Urinary, CNS, tachycardia
Isoprenaline	Beta receptor agonist (chronotropic and inotropic)	Ventricular bradycardia	Ventricular arrhythmias

NB: QT interval reflects action potential.
* = AV node effect; ** = Effects on atrioventricular accessory pathways; † = Ventricular effects.

Table 2: *Antiarrhythmic medication: dosages*

Agent	Oral	IV	Indications	Maintenance
Adenosine		Rapid bolus, 3, 6, 12 mg	AV re-entry tachycardia	
Amiodarone	Up to 1200 mg (divided doses)	300 mg 1st hour. 900 mg over next 23 hours. Central vein infusion	Atrial and ventricular arrhythmias	Oral 100–400 mg per day at night
Atropine		600 to 1200 mcg boluses	SA bradycardia	
Azimilide	100–125 mg per day		Atrial fibrillation	
Beta-blockers				
Esmolol		50–300 mg/kg /min, short-acting	Slowing down atrial and ventricular rhythms	
Metoprolol	25–100 mg twice daily	1–2 mg/min up to 15 mg	Slowing down atrial arrhythmias	25–100 mg bd
Propranolol	20, 40, 80 mg 8-hourly	1 mg/min, maximum 10 mg	As metoprolol	80–320 mg od oral
Bretylium tosylate		5–10 mg/kg over 10–30 min in 50 ml of dextrose saline	Resistant VF to DC shock	
Digitalis	Digitalising dose 1.5 mg in divided doses	0.5 mg slow, (IM 0.5 mg)	Atrial arrhythmias	0.125–0.25 mg od
Diltiazem	60–360 mg tds	0.25 mg/kg over 2 min	Atrial arrhythmias	Oral 60–300 mg od IV 5–15 mg/hour
Disopyramide	300 mg loading	100–150 mg over 5–10 min	Atrial and ventricular arrhythmias	IV and oral 800 mg per day
Flecainide	50–200 mg a day	1–2 mg/kg over 10 min	Atrial and ventricular arrhythmias	Oral 50–100 mg bd
Isoprenaline		0.5–10 mcg/min diluted	Complete heart block, slow ventricular rhythm	
Lignocaine		100 mg bolus	Ventricular arrhythmias	IV 1–4 mg/min
Mexiletine	200 mg 8-hourly	100–250 mg over 5–10 min	Ventricular arrhythmias	IV 0.5–1 mg/min oral 200 mg 8-hourly
Phenytoin	400–600 mg daily	10–15 mg/kg over 1 hour	Ventricular arrhythmias	Oral 400–600 mg per day
Procainamide	1 g stat then 500 mg 3-hourly	100 mg over 2 min	Ventricular arrhythmias	

Table 2: Continued

Agent	Oral	IV	Indications	Maintenance
Propafenone	150–300 mg		Atrial and ventricular arrhythmias	Oral 150 mg 8-hourly up to 1200 mg per day
Quinidine sulphate	300 mg 4-hourly up to 2 g per day		Atrial arrhythmias	Oral 300–600 mg per day
Sotalol	40 mg–80 mg bd	100 mg in 5 min	Atrial and ventricular arrhythmias	Oral 40–80 mg bd, up to 640 mg per day
Tocainide	300 mg stat		Ventricular arrhythmias	Oral 300–600 mg 8-hourly
Verapamil	40–120 mg up to 120 mg tds	5–10 mg over 5–10 min	Atrial arrhythmias, right ventricular outflow and fascicular VT	Oral 40–120 mg per day up to 120 mg 8-hourly IV 1 mg/min to 10 mg

NB: Dosages listed are for adults only.

Index

Page numbers in *italics* refer to figures or ECGs.

AAI pacing 189
ablation
   AV node 148
   pulmonary vein 149
   re-entry circuit 148
accelerated idioventricular rhythm 157
accessory pathways
   atrioventricular re-entrant
      tachycardia 113
   pre-excitation conduction 97-104,
      97-103
Adams–Stokes attacks 73
adenosine 228, 229
   stress testing 58
AIDS-related myocarditis 183
alcohol consumption *134*
alcoholic dilated cardiomyopathy *175*
amiodarone 228, 229
   in atrial fibrillation 146-7
   DC cardioversion and 204
   dose 229
   for ventricular premature beats 151
   in ventricular tachycardia 159
amyloid 176
aneurysm, left ventricular *13, 20, 210*
angina
   exercise/stress testing 54-60, *55-6*
   at rest (variant, Prinzmetal) *47-8*, 60
   unstable *51-2*, 60
      ischaemic changes *23-5*
      stress testing *58*
anterior hemiblock (left) 7, *7*, 80, *81*
antiarrhythmic agents 228-30
antibiotics, prophylactic 202
anticoagulation
   in atrial fibrillation 146, 147

   for DC cardioversion 147, 204
aortic stenosis
   left atrial hypertrophy *165-6*
   left bundle branch block *85-6*
   stress testing *56*, 57
arrhythmias 105-58
   on exercise/stress testing 57
   supraventricular (SVT) 105-49
   ventricular 105, 149-59
arrhythmogenic right ventricular
      dysplasia 157
aspirin 146
athlete's heart *94, 211*
atria
   abnormal activity 116-47
   electrical impulses 3
atrial bigeminy 105, *108*
atrial defibrillators, implantable 148
atrial ectopic beats (premature beats,
      APBs) 105-6, *106-9*, 113
atrial fibrillation 132-47, *133-46,
      205-7, 220*
   DC cardioversion 202
   lone 132
   management 146-9
   pacemaker insertion *198-9*
atrial flutter 120, *120-32, 197, 215*
   atypical (type II) 120
   DC cardioversion 202
   drug therapy 147
   typical (type I) 120
atrial parasystole 106
atrial tachycardia 118-19
   drug therapy 147
   multifocal 119
   unifocal 118-19, *119*

atrial trigeminy 105
atrioventricular (AV) block 68-78
  first degree 68, *68-70, 209*
  management 78
  predisposing conditions 78
  second degree 71, *71-2, 76, 208*
  third degree (complete) 73, *73-7,
    205, 208*
      atrial fibrillation with 132
      congenital 78
      pacing *192-7*
      post-infarction *30*
atrioventricular (AV) dissociation 73,
    116, 151, *208*
atrioventricular (AV) junctional
    tachycardia 116, *116-18*
atrioventricular (AV) node 1, *1*
  ablation 148
atrioventricular (AV) sequential pacing
    188
atrioventricular nodal re-entrant
    (AVNR) tachycardia 110-12, 147
  common 110, *110-12*
  uncommon 112, *112-13*
atrioventricular re-entrant tachycardia
    113, *114-15*
  antidromic 113
  orthodromic 113
atropine 78, 228, 229
  DC cardioversion and 203, 204
  stress echocardiography 60
augmented leads 2, 6, *6*
autoimmune disorders 177
AV, *see* atrioventricular
axis, electrical 5-7
azimilide 228, 229

beta-blockers
  doses 229-33
  stress testing and 54
  in supraventricular tachycardia 147,
    148, 159
bicycle testing 54
bifascicular block 81, *83, 84, 137, 206*
biventricular pacing 189
blood pressure, exercise/stress testing
    and 57
bradycardia
  asymptomatic 188

  sinus 64, *64, 66*
  symptomatic 188
  tilt test causing 189
bretylium 228, 229
broad complex tachycardias 156
  see also QRS complex, broad
Bruce, RA 62
Bruce protocol 54
Brugada, P 159
Brugada syndrome 158
bundle branch block 78-81, *82-94*
  rate-related *93-4*
  see also left bundle branch block;
    right bundle branch block
bundle of His 1, *1*, 78
bundle of Kent 97

caffeine consumption *106-7*
captured beats 151
cardiac failure, congestive 146, 151
cardiogenic shock 61, 204
cardiomyopathies 169-76
  definition 169
  dilated 151, 173, *174-5*
  hypertrophic (obstructive) (HOCM)
    169, *170-3, 217*
  ischaemic 175
  primary 169-76
  restrictive 176
  secondary 176
cardioversion
  DC, *see* DC cardioversion
  medical 146-7
cardioverter/defibrillators, implantable
    (ICDs) 202-3
carotid massage 95
carotid sinus syndrome 95, *95-6*
Chagas' disease 183
chest pain 54
chronotropic incompetence 65
cocaine 185
conducting system, heart 1, *1*, 78, *78*
  surgical trauma *91-3*
conduction impairment 63-104
  on exercise/stress testing 57
  pre-excitation 97-104, *97-103*
coronary artery
  dissection *50, 51*
  spasm *47-8*, 60

coronary heart disease, *see* ischaemic (coronary) heart disease

DC cardioversion 147, 159, 203-4
  emergency 204
  patients with pacemakers 202
  risks 203-4
  in ventricular tachycardia 159, 203, 204
DDD pacing 189
'dead window' 10
defibrillators
  external 203
  implantable atrial 148
  internal 203
delta waves, in WPW syndrome 97, *97-103*, 113
depolarisation, muscle *2*
diabetes mellitus 54
digitalis 228, 229
digoxin
  stress testing and 54
  for SVT arrhythmias 147
  toxicity 68, 183, *183-5*
diltiazem 228, 229
dipyridamole stress test 58
disopyramide 228, 229
dobutamine stress testing 60
dofetilide 147, 148
driving, by patients with pacemakers or ICDs 203
drugs
  causing ECG changes 183-5
  prolonging QT interval 104, 158
  regimen tables 228-30
  stress testing and 54
Duchenne muscular dystrophy 176

echocardiography, stress 60
Einthoven, W 8
Einthoven triangle *5*
electrical alternans 179, *191*
electrical axis 5-7
electrical impulses, cardiac 1-2, *1*
  topography 3-5
electrodes
  ECG, positioning 2-3, *2*
  pacemaker, problems 201
electrolyte disturbances 185

electrophysiological study (EPS) 159
emboli
  coronary *46*
  systemic 146, 203-4
ergometry, bicycle 54
esmolol 147
exercise ECG/stress testing 54-60, *55-6, 216*
  in bundle branch block 80
  echocardiography 60
  false positives 57, *58*
  nuclear (isotope) 58-9, *59*
  other ECG abnormalities 57
exit block 201

fascicular ventricular tachycardia 157
flecainide 228, 229
Friedreich's ataxia 174
fusion beats 151
F waves 120

heart block, *see* atrioventricular (AV) block
heart rate
  delayed decrease, on exercise testing 57
  turbulence 62
  variability 61
hemiblocks 80, *81*
heparin 147, 204
hexaxial system 6, *6*
hibernating myocardium 61
His, W 8
Holter, NJ 159
hypercalcaemia 185
hyperkalaemia 185
hypermagnesaemia 185
hypertrophy 161-68
hypocalcaemia 185
hypokalaemia 185
hypomagnesaemia 185
hypothermia 185
hysteresis 201

identity cards 187
implantable atrial defibrillators 148
implantable cardioverter/defibrillators (ICDs) 202-3

inferior hemiblock (right axis deviation) 7, 7, 80, *81*
ischaemic (coronary) heart disease 9-62, *210*
  atrial fibrillation *133, 135, 139-42*
  conduction impairment *89-90*
  exercise ECG/stress testing, *see* exercise ECG/stress testing
  ischaemic cardiomyopathy *175*
  ventricular premature beats 151
  see also angina; myocardial infarction; myocardial ischaemia
isoprenaline 78, 228, 229
isotope stress exercise testing 58-9, *59*

Jervel-Lange-Nielsen syndrome 104, 158
junctional tachycardia 116, *116-18*

left atrial hypertrophy (LAH) 164, *165-8, 170*
  causes 164
left axis deviation (LAD, left anterior hemiblock) 7, 7, 80, *81*
left bundle 1, 78
left bundle branch block (LBBB) 79-80, *84-90, 207*
  myocardial infarction and *29*, 80
left rabbit ear 156
left ventricle
  aneurysm *13, 20, 210*
  depolarisation *6*
left ventricular hypertrophy (LVH) 161, *162-4, 173, 177*
  causes 161
  strain pattern 161, *162-4, 167, 216, 220*
lignocaine 151, 159, 228, 229
limb leads 2, 5, *5*, 6
lithium 185
Lown-Ganong-Levine syndrome 103, *103*

magnesium, for prolonged QT interval 158
'Maze' operation 148
metabolic disturbances 185
metoprolol 229
mexiletine 228, 229

mobile telephones, pacemakers and 202
Mobitz I second degree heart block 71, *71*
Mobitz II second degree heart block 71, *72, 76, 208*
muscle depolarisation *2*
muscular dystrophy, Duchenne 176
myocardial infarction
  anterior 10, *10-25, 222*
  anterolateral 10, *35-6, 209*
  anteroseptal 10, *13-20, 210*
  exercise/stress testing and 57
  inferior 26, *26-30, 37-42*
  left bundle branch block and *29*, 80
  non Q wave, *see* non Q wave (subendocardial) infarction
  other ECG indices 61-2
  progression of changes after 32, *32-53*
  Q wave (transmural, full thickness) 10-31
  silent *43*
  true posterior 30, *31, 218*
  ventricular premature beats after 151
  ventricular tachycardia after 156
myocardial ischaemia
  atrial fibrillation causing *140-1*
  clinical features 54
  silent *49*, 54
  see also angina
myocarditis 182-3
  viral *88*, 182, *182*
myopotential inhibition 201
myotonic dystrophy 176
myxoedema 176

nomenclature
  ECG 3, *3*
  pacemaker 188
non Q wave (subendocardial) infarction 9, *9, 217-18, 220-1*
  progression over time 32, *32-5, 38-9*
normal ECG recording *3*
nuclear (isotope) stress exercise testing 58-9, *59*

overdrive suppression test 159
overpacing 202

pacemakers 187–202, *190–200*
    complications 189, 201, *221*
    driving and 203
    external 202
    general precautions 202
    nomenclature 188
    permanent 187–201
        failure 201, *219*
        follow up 201
        indications *67*, 78
    temporary 201–2
        indications 78, 202
    types in use 189
    see also specific types of pacing
pacemaker syndrome 189
pericarditis 179–81
    acute 179, *179–81*
    chronic 181, *181*
phenothiazines 184
phenytoin 228, 229
P mitrale 164, *165*
polyarteritis nodosa (PAN) 177
P pulmonale 168, *175*
precordial leads 3
pre-excitation conduction 97–104,
    97–103
PR interval 3, *3*
    prolonged 68, 71
    short, in WPW syndrome 97,
        97–103
Prinzmetal, M 62
procainamide 228, 229
propafenone 147, 228
propranolol 229
pulmonary vein ablation 149
Purkinje, JE 8
Purkinje system 1, *1*
P waves 3, *3, 4*
    in atrial parasystole 106
    in atrial tachycardia 118, *119*
    in junctional tachycardia *116–18*
    premature 105
    in right atrial hypertrophy 168
    in ventricular tachycardia 151, *156*

QRS complex 3, *3, 4*

    broad (wide) 156
        in bundle branch block 79
        in supraventricular arrhythmias
            105, 113
        in ventricular arrhythmias 149,
            151
    distortion of terminal, with reduced
        S waves 53
    duration 3
    'M'-shaped 79, 80
    narrow 105, 116
QT dispersion 61
QT interval *3*
    normal 3
    prolonged 104, 158
        acquired 158
        congenital 158
quinidine 204, 228, 230
    syncope 148
    toxicity 183
Q waves
    abnormal 53
    in anterior infarction 10, *12*, *17–18*
    in inferior infarction *27*, *28–30*
    'positional' *213–14*
    progression over time 32
    in true posterior infarction *31*
Q wave (transmural, full thickness)
    infarction 10–31
    progression over time 32, *32–53*

rabbit ear, left 156
re-entry circuit 97
    ablation 148
re-entry supraventricular tachycardia
    103, *103*, 110–13
rheumatic fever 183
rhythm disturbances, *see* arrhythmias
right atrial hypertrophy (RAH) 168,
    175
right axis deviation (RAD, inferior
    hemiblock) 7, *7*, 80, *81*
right bundle 1, 78
right bundle branch block (RBBB) 79,
    79, 80, *82–4*, 206, *211*
    post-infarction *13*, *52*, *53*
    post-surgical *93*
right ventricular dysplasia,
    arrhythmogenic 157

right ventricular hypertrophy (RVH)
161, 177, *206*
causes 161
strain pattern 161
right ventricular outflow tract
tachycardia 157
Romano-Ward syndrome 104, 158
R waves
absent *43*
dominant, in true posterior
infarction 30, *31*
in Friedreich's ataxia 176
reduced progression
in anterior infarction *16, 21*
changes over time *34, 35-6, 52*
over precordial leads 53

sarcoidosis 176, *177*
scintigraphy (nuclear stress exercise
testing) 58-9, *59*
scleroderma 177
Senning, A 204
septum, interventricular
activation 4
hypertrophy 161
sick sinus syndrome 65, *145, 190-1*
silent myocardial infarction *43*
silent myocardial ischaemia *49*, 54
sinoatrial arrest 65, *65-7*
in healthy young adult *94*
sinoatrial block 65, *66, 67*
in healthy young adult *94*
sinoatrial disease 64-5, *65-7*
sinoatrial (SA) node 1, *1*
sinoatrial tachycardia 65
sinus arrhythmia 63, *63*
sinus bradycardia 64, *64, 66*
sinus node recovery time 159
sinus tachycardia 64
sodium concentrations, altered 185
sotalol 228-30
stress testing, *see* exercise ECG/stress
testing
stroke 146
ST segment *3*
changes during exercise *56*, 57, *58*
depression 62
in anterior Q wave infarction
13-14, 17

exercise/stress testing 54, *55-6,
215*
in inferior Q wave infarction *30*
in non Q wave infarction 9, *9*
progression over time *40, 41-2,
44-5, 49*
with T wave inversion 53
elevation 62, *213, 214*
in anterior infarction *11-13, 17,
20, 21, 24*
exercise/stress testing 57
in inferior infarction *26*
in non Q wave infarction 9, *9*
in pericarditis 179, *179-80*
progression over time 32, *34-5,
37-8, 47-8*
stunned myocardium 61
subendocardial infarction, *see* non Q
wave (subendocardial) infarction
sudden death 158
in hypertrophic cardiomyopathy 169
prolonged QT interval and 104
supraventricular arrhythmias (SVT)
105-49
emergency cardioversion 204
exercise/stress testing and 57
mechanical management 148-9
pharmacological management 147-8
prevention 148
re-entry mechanism 110-13
supraventricular re-entry tachycardia
103, *103*, 110-13, 147
surgery
conducting system trauma *91-3*
in supraventricular arrhythmias 148
syncope
carotid sinus 95, *95-6*
long QT interval 104
quinidine 228
tilt testing 189, *199-200*
syndrome X 60-1
systemic lupus erythematosus (SLE) 177

tachy/brady (sick sinus) syndrome 65,
145, 190-1
tachycardia
atrial, *see* atrial tachycardia
atrioventricular nodal re-entrant
110-12

atrioventricular re-entrant 113,
    114-15, 147
  broad complex 156
  junctional 116, *116-18*
  pacemaker-induced *221*
  right ventricular outflow tract 157
  sinus 64
  ventricular, *see* ventricular
    tachycardia
technetium testing 58
thallium stress testing 58, *59*
thrombolysin therapy 27, *41-2*
tilt test 189, *199-200*, *215*
tocainide 228, 230
torsade de pointes 104, 151, 157, *157*
transient ischaemic attacks (TIAs)
    190-1
treadmill testing 54
tremor *212*
triaxial system 5, *6*
tricyclic antidepressants 184
trifascicular block *68*, 81, *83*, 87
tuberculous pericarditis *180*
T waves *3*, 5
  in hypertrophic cardiomyopathy
    170-1, *172*
  inversion
    in anterior infarction *12*, *16*, *19*,
        23
    exercise/stress testing *56*
    in inferior infarction *28*, *30*
    in non Q wave infarction 9
    in pericarditis 179
    progression over time 32, *35-6*,
        44-7
    ST segment depression with 53
  new, tall and peaked 53
  in WPW syndrome *99*, *102*

Uhl's syndrome 157
U wave *3*

VDD pacing 189, *192*, *196*, *209*, *219*
ventricles
  activation 5
  electrical impulses 4-5

ventricular arrhythmias 105, 149-59
  exercise/stress testing and 57
ventricular bigeminy *149*, 150
ventricular couplets 150, *150*
ventricular extrasystoles (premature
    beats, VPBs) 112, 113, 149-51
  management 151
  multifocal 149
  preceding ventricular tachycardia
    156
  unifocal 149, *211*
ventricular fibrillation (VF) 151, 158
  DC cardioversion 203, 204
  implantable
    cardioverter/defibrillators 202-3
ventricular late potentials 61
ventricular parasystole 150
ventricular salvo 150
ventricular tachycardia (VT) 151-8,
    152-6, *218*
  artefactual *212*
  causes 156
  fascicular 157
  monomorphic/polymorphic 151
  slow 157
  symptoms 158
  treatment 159, 202-3, 204
  types 157
  in WPW syndrome 97, *102*
ventricular trigeminy 150
verapamil 147, 228, 230
viral myocarditis *88*, 182, *182*
Von Koellitzer, A 8
VVI pacing 189, *191*, *193*, *194*,
    198-9, *207*

Waller, AD 8
wandering pacemaker 63
warfarin
  in atrial fibrillation 146, 147
  for DC cardioversion 204
Wenckebach phenomenon 71, *71*
Wolff-Parkinson-White (WPW)
    syndrome 97, *97-103*, 113
  drug therapy 228
  intermittent *101*